NEUROINFLAMMATION IN DISEASE

RISK FACTORS, MANAGEMENT AND OUTCOMES

Neuroscience Research Progress

NEUROSCIENCE RESEARCH PROGRESS

NEUROINFLAMMATION IN DISEASE

RISK FACTORS, MANAGEMENT AND OUTCOMES

REBECCA K. DAWSON
EDITOR

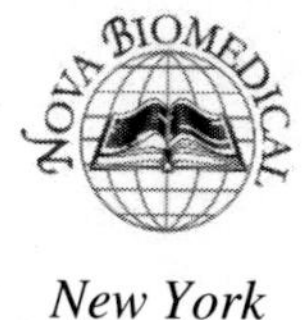

New York

NOTICE TO THE READER

Library of Congress Cataloging-in-Publication Data

Library of Congress Control Number: 2015945231

ISBN: 978-1-63483-389-9

Published by Nova Science Publishers, Inc. † New York

Contents

Preface

In this book, the link between the modifiable risk factors of neuro-degenerative diseases and chronic neuroinflammation are examined, thus highlighting that controlling risk factors is a valid approach for managing neurodegnerative diseases in which neuroinflammation contributes to the disease progression. The mechanisms of inhibition of neuroinflammation by EST and ERAs are discussed, as well as the neuroprotective roles of EST and ERAs in multiple sclerosis, Alzheimer's disease, Parkinson's disease and epilepsy. The final chapter focuses on the dynamics of progression in MS patients, and the disease process within contexts of proinflammatory reactivity and interactivity.

Chapter I – Alzheimer's disease (AD), Parkinson's disease (PD), and amyotrophic lateral sclerosis (ALS) are three common neurodegenerative diseases, which increasingly contribute to morbidity and mortality worldwide. Although each of these diseases is characterized by a unique pathology, they all share neuroinflammation as a common underlying feature. Recent evidence indicates that neuroinflammation is initially triggered by pathological processes associated with specific diseases; however, it becomes chronic and can contribute to disease progression. Chronic neuroinflammation is generally characterized by dysregulated activation of the immune cells of the brain, the microglia. This process, which has been termed microgliosis, can lead to collateral damage of the surrounding neurons, due to the non-specific nature of the innate immune system responses, and contribute to the neurodegeneration observed in diseases of the central nervous system, such as AD, PD and ALS. Several studies have identified diets high in polyunsaturated fats, sedentary lifestyle, as well as lifestyle-induced diseases, such as type 2 diabetes mellitus (T2DM), as risk factors for developing AD, PD and ALS. Research has shown that the same risk factors can also contribute to microgliosis and help sustain the subsequent neuroinflammatory environment, which may drive the progression of these specific diseases. It has been suggested that altering the aforementioned modifiable risk factors and making certain lifestyle changes could reduce the risk of developing these diseases. In the following chapter, we will describe the link between the modifiable risk factors of neurodegenerative diseases and chronic neuroinflammation, thus highlighting that controlling risk factors is a valid approach for managing neuro-degenerative diseases in which neuroinflammation contributes to the disease progression.

Chapter II – There are multiple connections between the central nervous system (CNS) and the immune system so as to regulate the innate immune responses for normal neurological functions in humans. Microglial cells play the most crucial role against wound or microbial infection and stimulate an array of secondary responses through astrocyte activation and recruitment of peripheral immune cells into the CNS. Estrogen receptor agonists (ERAs) can modulate the activity of many cell types involved in the immune response in the CNS. Recent studies confirmed that ERAs could modulate different inflammatory processes in animal models of human CNS diseases such as multiple sclerosis (MS), epilepsy, Parkinson's disease (PD), Alzheimer disease (AD), and spinal cord injury (SCI). Recent studies demonstrated that ERAs can control activation of microglia, migration of blood-derived monocytes to the infected area, and inhibition of expression of pro-inflammatory cytokines (IL-1β and TNF-α) in the CNS. Neuroprotective effects of ERAs are mainly mediated by estrogen receptor alpha (ERα) and ER beta (ERβ), which are a member of the nuclear hormone family of intracellular receptors. ERs are expressed in various cell types of the immune system, including macrophages, microglia, and T cells. The exact mechanisms of modulation of different neuroinflammatory pathways in the CNS are not completely known. Research on ERAs and different CNS disorders still remains in its early stage but several studies have indicated promising therapeutic effects of ERAs in delaying the onset neuroinflammation and thus symptomatic recovery in some CNS disorders. This book chapter will highlight some recent developments on mechanisms of action and therapeutic effects of ERAs in prevention of neurodegeneration and neuroinflammation in different CNS disorders.

Chapter III – Dynamics of progression in MS patients are indices of reference of an essential establishment of the disease process within contexts of proinflammatory reactivity and interactivity of an activated endothelial cell bed that perfuses the CNS parenchyma. The specific character of the activation of endothelial cells incorporates correlates of dynamic turnover and loss of myelin in plaques that persistently expand in a relapsing/recurring manner. The inclusive phenomenon of endothelial cell response and injury calls, into operative distribution, lesions that comprise both edema and ischemia within the individual MS plaque. It is such phenomenon of inclusive establishment of the initial microvascular injury that persists in terms of specific activation states of the endothelial cells lining post-capillary venules and capillaries of the cerebrovasculature.

Chapter I

An Interplay between Neuroinflammation and Modifiable Risk Factors of Alzheimer's Disease, Parkinson's Disease and Amyotrophic Lateral Sclerosis

Stephanie M. Schindler, Lindsay J. Spielman,
Caitlin B. Pointer, Wyatt T. Slattery, Ekta Bajwa,
Jordan A. McKenzie, Jessica R. Lowry
and Andis Klegeris[1,*]
Department of Biology,
University of British Columbia Okanagan Campus,
Kelowna, British Columbia, Canada

* Corresponding Author Address: Andis Klegeris, DPhil; Department of Biology, University of British Columbia Okanagan Campus, Kelowna, British Columbia, V1V 1V7 CANADA; andis.klegeris@ubc.ca; (P) 250-807-9557; (F) 250-807-8830

Abstract

Alzheimer's disease (AD), Parkinson's disease (PD), and amyotrophic lateral sclerosis (ALS) are three common neurodegenerative diseases, which increasingly contribute to morbidity and mortality worldwide. Although each of these diseases is characterized by a unique pathology, they all share neuroinflammation as a common underlying feature. Recent evidence indicates that neuroinflammation is initially triggered by pathological processes associated with specific diseases; however, it becomes chronic and can contribute to disease progression. Chronic neuroinflammation is generally characterized by dysregulated activation of the immune cells of the brain, the microglia. This process, which has been termed microgliosis, can lead to collateral damage of the surrounding neurons, due to the non-specific nature of the innate immune system responses, and contribute to the neurodegeneration observed in diseases of the central nervous system, such as AD, PD and ALS.

Several studies have identified diets high in polyunsaturated fats, sedentary lifestyle, as well as lifestyle-induced diseases, such as type 2 diabetes mellitus (T2DM), as risk factors for developing AD, PD and ALS. Research has shown that the same risk factors can also contribute to microgliosis and help sustain the subsequent neuroinflammatory environment, which may drive the progression of these specific diseases. It has been suggested that altering the aforementioned modifiable risk factors and making certain lifestyle changes could reduce the risk of developing these diseases. In the following chapter, we will describe the link between the modifiable risk factors of neurodegenerative diseases and chronic neuroinflammation, thus highlighting that controlling risk factors is a valid approach for managing neurodegenerative diseases in which neuroinflammation contributes to the disease progression.

1. Non-Modifiable Risk Factors of Neurodegenerative Diseases

Alzheimer's disease (AD), Parkinson's disease (PD), and amyotrophic lateral sclerosis (ALS) are three neurodegenerative diseases, which increasingly contribute to morbidity and mortality, affecting over 50 million people worldwide [1-3]. Numerous studies have attempted to describe the causes and factors associated with the risk for the development and progression of these three diseases, and have identified a number of potential non-modifiable risk factors including, genetics and exposure to certain environmental factors [4-9], as well as some modifiable risk factors, such as diets high in polyunsaturated fatty acids (PUFAs), sedentary lifestyle, and lifestyle-induced diseases (Figure 1) [10-12]. In this chapter we will first describe the non-modifiable risk factors for AD, PD and ALS, followed by a discussion of the modifiable risk factors.

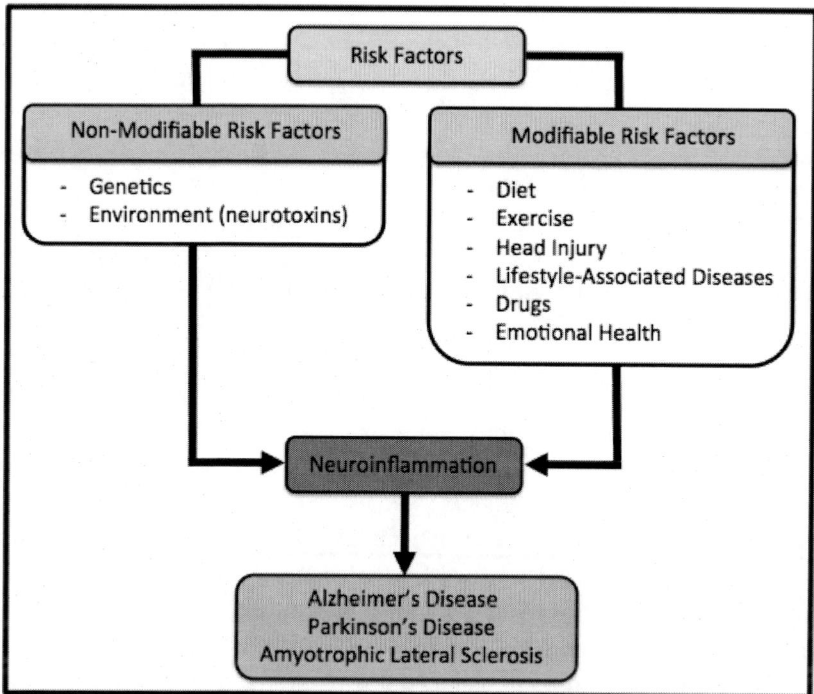

Figure 1. Non-modifiable and modifiable risk factors for neuroinflammation, which is the common link between a number of neurodegenerative diseases including AD, PD and ALS.

Over the past years, genome-wide association studies have helped to considerably increase our understanding of the genetics of AD, PD and ALS, and have also uncovered many genetic variants that confer increased risk for these three neurodegenerative diseases [13-16]. The most commonly studied gene mutations associated with the familial AD are located in the genes encoding the amyloid precursor protein (APP) and the presenilins 1 and 2; they lead to a more active amyloidogenic pathway and subsequent increased production of amyloid-beta protein (Aβ) [17, 18]. Apolipoprotein E (APOE) is the most common genetic risk factor for the late-onset sporadic AD. The APOE gene contains three main polymorphisms, ε2, ε3, and ε4, of which ε4 was found to be associated with increased risk of developing late-onset AD [18, 19]. In the presence of one ε4 allele the relative risk (RR) for progression from mild cognitive impairment (MCI) to AD was 1.84, which increased to 3.02 in cases with APOEε4/ε4 [19].

PD and ALS have also been shown to have genetic components. For example, mutations in the α-synuclein gene can result in the overexpression of the α-synuclein protein in the brain leading to the accumulation and aggregation of the protein into Lewy bodies, which are the pathological hallmarks of PD [7, 20, 21]. Furthermore, these mutations may raise the lifetime risk of developing PD by 25-30% [22]. The risk for developing ALS has also been associated with mutations in several genes, including superoxide dismutase (SOD) 1 [6, 23]. SOD1 protein is an antioxidant that converts superoxide radicals to hydrogen peroxide. The mutation results in a toxic gain of function for this protein acquiring prion-like properties and the ability to form toxic aggregates, which have shown to be important in the pathology of ALS [23].

In addition to genetic risk factors, the role of the environment as a potential risk factor for AD, PD and ALS has gained recognition. Specifically, the effects of exposure to neurotoxic metals such as lead through contaminated drinking water on the onset of AD, PD and ALS have been investigated [8, 9, 24]. Despite few epidemiological studies showing no direct association between lead exposure and development of AD [25], several experimental studies have demonstrated a potential link between lead exposure and AD development [26-28]. For example, monkeys exposed to lead at a young age had enhanced APP expression leading to a significant increase in Aβ plaque load [26]. Similar results were obtained *in vitro* using differentiated SH-SY5Y neuronal cells. Incubation of SH-SY5Y cells with lead augmented APP expression, Aβ secretion, as well as decreased the expression and protein levels of an Aβ degrading enzyme [27, 28].

Chronic exposure to lead is also associated with an increased risk for developing PD, with one study recording a two-fold increase in PD risk for individuals in the highest quartile for lifetime lead exposure relative to the lowest quartile [29]. Experimental studies revealed that lead decreased dopamine release and the expression of the dopamine D1 receptor in rats [30]. Lead exposure also caused aggregation of α-synuclein [31], which could provide an explanation for PD-like symptoms observed in affected individuals.

Kamel et al. [32] conducted a study to assess blood and bone lead levels in 109 ALS patients and 256 control patients. They found that ALS was associated with elevated levels of lead in both blood and bone; showing a 1.9

fold increase in risk for each μg/dl increment in blood level. Moreover, the risk increased 2.3-3.6 fold for each doubling of lead concentration in the bone [32]. The authors went on to suggest that mobilization of lead from bone into the blood may occur during the acute onset of ALS. A more recent meta-analysis estimated a 5% increase in the risk of developing ALS in individuals with a history of lead exposure [33].

In addition to lead, exposure to other environmental pollutants, such as pesticides have been linked to an increased susceptibility for the development of select neurodegenerative diseases later on in life [8]. Moreover, epigenetic DNA modifications, including DNA methylation and histone acetylation may be caused by maternal exposure to certain environmental stimuli during critical periods of fetal development [8]. These epigenetic changes related to environmental factors have been suggested to be involved in neuro-degenerative diseases [23, 34].

2. Neuroinflammation in Neurodegenerative Diseases

AD, PD and ALS are all characterized by unique pathologies; however they also share a common underlying feature: neuroinflammation, which is characterized by the dysregulated activation of the immune cells of the brain, the microglia [35, 36]. Microglia are responsible for mounting an immune response to a variety of insults, including infections, trauma, toxins and a variety of other stimuli [37, 38]. Activation of microglia leads to their morphological and functional changes, which result in a transformation from a resting (ramified) phenotype to a phagocytic (amoeboid) phenotype aimed at eliminating the insult (Figure 2) [39, 40]. These changes also include increased expression of cell membrane receptors, such as major histocompatibility complex (MHC)-II and macrophage antigen complex (Mac)-1 [39], as well as increased release of inflammatory mediators, such as cytokines (e.g., interleukin (IL)-1β and tumor necrosis factor (TNF)-α), chemokines (e.g., monocyte chemotactic protein (MCP)-1), nitric oxide (NO) and reactive oxygen species (ROS) [41, 42]. In addition, microglia release neurotrophic factors, such as brain-derived neurotrophic factor (BDNF), neurotrophin (NT)-3 and NT-4, which are essential to neuronal survival and re-establishing homeostasis in the brain [35, 41]. Therefore, in general, this acute neuroinflammatory response is beneficial, as it contributes to removing or repairing damaged tissue.

In contrast, chronic neuroinflammation is often self-perpetuating and persists long after the initial insult has been cleared. In this chronic inflammatory state, microglial activation progresses to microgliosis and is accompanied by the increased and sustained release of the pro-inflammatory mediators. Due to the non-specific nature of the pro-inflammatory response, microgliosis can lead to collateral damage to the surrounding neurons and may contribute to the neurodegeneration observed. AD, PD and ALS have all been shown to be associated with chronic neuroinflammation, microgliosis and elevated levels of pro-inflammatory cytokines, which can modify disease progression [38-40, 43-45]. Microglial activation in AD and PD is primarily caused by the presence of pathology-associated molecules: Aβ [46] and α-synuclein [47], respectively; while in ALS the exact molecule(s) responsible for triggering microglial activation remain unclear. A mutated form of the SOD1 protein has been suggested to play a role in initiating the inflammatory response [48, 49].

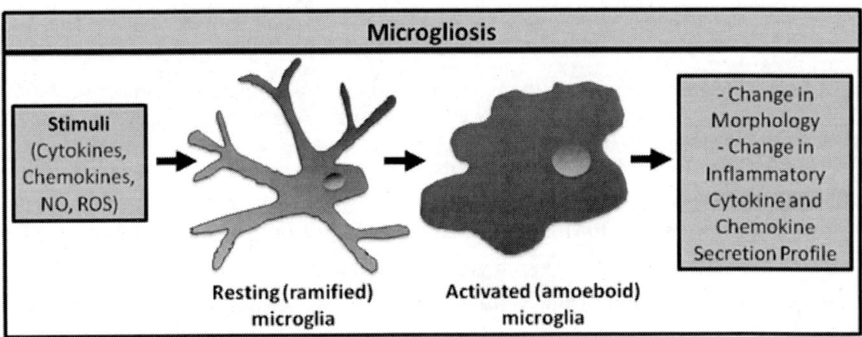

Figure 2. Microglial activation (microgliosis) induced by pro-inflammatory mediators such as cytokines leads to morphological and physiological changes of the cells.

Several studies have demonstrated that Aβ can induce microgliosis using rodent and human microglia cell lines [50-52] as well as primary cells [53-56], which was accompanied by the abnormal expression of cytokines, chemokines and other pro-inflammatory molecules. Stimulation of human THP-1 monocytic cells (a microglia model) with Aβ led to activation of the pro-inflammatory mitogen activated protein kinase (MAPK) and nuclear factor-kappa B (NF-κB) pathways, which resulted in the increased expression of TNF-α and IL-1β [51]. Furthermore, conditioned media from the Aβ-stimulated THP-1 cells induced TNF-α-dependent neuronal apoptosis [51]. Similar results were obtained with primary human microglia upon treatment with Aβ [54-56]. Gene array analysis and quantitative polymerase chain reaction (qPCR) showed upregulation of IL-8, MCP-1, IL-1β and TNF-α in microglia, which supported the hypothesis that the interaction of microglia and Aβ promotes inflammation, due to the induction of several pro-inflammatory and potentially neurotoxic cytokines [55].

Similar findings have been obtained in studies related to PD pathogenesis, which demonstrated the increased presence of activated microglia and inflammatory mediators (TNF-α, IL-1β, IL-6 and interferon (IFN)-γ) in the brains and cerebral spinal fluid (CSF) of PD patients [57-61]. Using [^{11}C](R)-PK11195, a positron emission tomography (PET) marker of peripheral benzodiazepine sites, which are selectively expressed by activated microglia, Gerhard et al. [58] demonstrated significantly increased binding of [^{11}C](R)-PK11195 in the pons, basal ganglia, and frontal and temporal cortical regions of PD brains [58]. These *in vivo* findings confirmed that activated microglia were associated with the pathological processes of PD. The role of α-synuclein as a microglial activator has been investigated using primary mouse and rat neuron-glia co-cultures, primary human microglia cultures, as well as *in vivo* PD mouse models [62-66]. Treatment of primary rat mesencephalic microglia with α-synuclein resulted in their activation characterized by the increased release of TNF-α, NO, ROS and prostaglandin (PG) E$_2$ [62, 67]. Furthermore, α-synuclein-induced toxicity to dopaminergic neurons was enhanced in the presence of microglia, while, conversely, the microglia-depleted cultures showed significantly decreased dopaminergic toxicity, which supported the essential role of microglia in PD neurodegeneration [62]. In addition, the researchers proposed that the microglia Mac-1 receptor was responsible for interacting with α-synuclein, thereby providing a potential target for regulating microglial activation.

Microglial activation and other inflammatory responses have also been demonstrated in ALS [23, 40, 44]. Neuroinflammation in individuals with ALS was evaluated using [(^{11})C](R)-PK11195 [68] and [(^{11})C]-PBR28 [69] PET scans. A significant increase in binding was found in the motor cortex, pons, dorsolateral prefrontal cortex and thalamus in the brains of ALS patients; thus supporting a role for activated microglia in ALS [68, 69]. Further evidence for the role of inflammation in ALS was provided by Kuhle et al. [70], who measured the levels of pro-inflammatory mediators in the CSF of ALS patients, and found that MCP-1 and IL-8 were significantly elevated compared to control brains. Furthermore, there was a trend towards a correlation between MCP-1 levels and survival time after diagnosis [70]. Spinal cord tissue from ALS patients also showed increased expression of activated dendritic (e.g., CD83, CD40) and monocytic (e.g., CD14, CD68) cell surface markers, as well as MCP-1 and macrophage-colony stimulating factor (M-CSF) [71]. Similar to the correlation observed by Kuhle et al. [67], patients who had a more rapid disease progression showed significantly increased expression of the activated immune cell markers [71], thus lending further support to the involvement of inflammatory responses in driving the progression of ALS.

Overall, the increasing evidence of the involvement of neuroinflammation in the development and progression of AD, PD and ALS (Figure 3), has led to research focused on microglia as attractive therapeutic targets in the treatment of these neurodegenerative diseases. However, rather than targeting microgliosis with the intention of reversing the existing neuroinflammatory state, a more effective strategy may be to prevent acute inflammation from progressing to microgliosis in the first place.

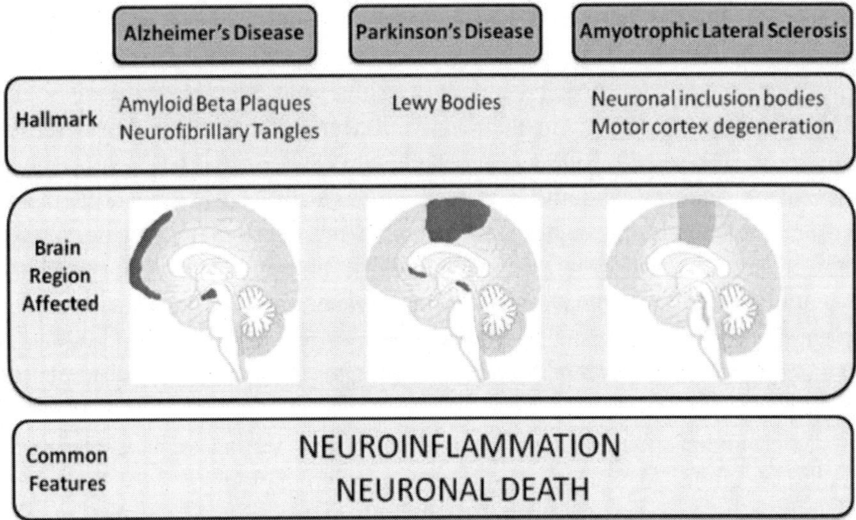

Figure 3. The hallmarks, affected brain regions and common underlying features of AD, PD and ALS.

3. Effects of Modifiable Risk Factors on Neuroinflammation

Several studies have identified diets high in PUFAs, sedentary lifestyle, as well as lifestyle-induced diseases, such as type 2 diabetes mellitus (T2DM), as risk factors for developing AD, PD and ALS. Research has shown that these risk factors can also contribute to microgliosis and help sustain the subsequent neuroinflammatory environment, thus driving the progression of specific diseases. It has been suggested that altering the aforementioned modifiable risk factors and making certain lifestyle changes could reduce the individual risk as well as the overall prevalence of these diseases. In the following sections, we will describe the link between the modifiable risk factors of neurodegenerative diseases and chronic neuroinflammation, thus highlighting controlling risk factors as a valid approach for managing neurodegenerative diseases in which neuroinflammation contributes to the disease progression.

3.1. Diet

In peripheral tissues, chronic inflammation has been shown to be a dynamic state, which can be modified through the control of specific risk factors; one such risk factor is habitual dietary consumption. Dietary components such as fiber, fatty acids, antioxidants, carotenoids, vitamins, and caffeine have all been shown to have a direct effect on specific aspects of inflammatory responses [72]. Discussed here are the ω-3 and ω-6 PUFAs, polyphenolic antioxidants, and the lifestyle drug, caffeine. These dietary factors have varying effects on central nervous system (CNS) inflammation including regulation of PG and leukotriene synthesis, pro-inflammatory mediator secretion, release of reactive nitrogen species (RNS), and functional status of the blood brain barrier (BBB).

PUFAs are essential to the human diet and constitute a wide range of fatty acids. Common ω-3 PUFAs include α-linolenic acid, eicosapentaenoic acid (EPA), and docosahexaenoic acid (DHA), whereas ω-6 PUFAs are primarily consumed as linoleic acid or arachidonic acid (AA) [73]. ω-3 and ω-6 PUFAs are implicated in the normal growth, development and function of mammalian cells, and are considered essential as they cannot be synthesized by the body [74, 75]. Additionally, PUFAs have been shown to have a regulatory role in the development and severity of neuroinflammation in neurodegenerative disease [76, 77]. Peterson et al.[78] demonstrated that rats fed diets supplemented with an elevated 7:1 ratio of AA to ω-3 PUFAs had a two-fold increase in the production of PGE_2; deregulation of this eicosanoid is associated with both chronic inflammation and the pathogenesis of neurodegenerative disorders, including AD [78, 79]. In contrast, dietary consumption of ω-3 PUFAs leads to metabolic products, such as EPA, which promote anti-inflammatory states both in the periphery and CNS [80, 81]. It has been found that consumption of long-chain ω-3 PUFAs decreases the amount of AA in the membranes of inflammatory cells and reduces the substrate availability for the synthesis of pro-inflammatory eicosanoids including PGE_2, thromboxane B_2, and leukotriene E_4 producing a whole-body anti-inflammatory effect [82, 83]. Furthermore, it has been identified that ω-3 PUFAs have eicosanoid-independent anti-inflammatory effects mediated through inhibition of the NF-κB pathway [82]. Since NF-κB plays a central role in a wide range of pro-inflammatory responses, inhibiting the activation of this transcription factor suppresses the expression of many pro-inflammatory cytokines, mediators, and enzymes such as inducible NO synthase (iNOS), TNF-α, IL-6, and IL-1β [74, 82, 84, 85]. Despite the opposing effects of ω-3 and ω-6 PUFA diet supplementation on inflammation, emphasis has been placed on the relative consumption of these compounds rather than their individual effects [74, 86]. Specifically, consumption of ω-3 and ω-6 PUFAs in a ratio of about 1:1 has been associated with the lowest levels of inflammatory markers [86]. In comparison, consumption of high ratios of ω-6 to ω-3 PUFAs, such as the ~16:1 ratio seen in Western diets, promotes the pathogenesis of cardiovascular disease, cancer, osteoporosis, inflammatory and autoimmune diseases [74]. With regard to controlling the intake of PUFAs as a modifiable risk factor, it was shown that neurological impairment in rats caused by a deficiency of dietary ω-3 was reversed upon reintroduction of ω-3 PUFAs to the diet [87]. Consistently with this observation, it was seen in a prospective study of 815 elderly individuals that dietary intake of ω-3 PUFAs through weekly consumption of fish reduced the incidence of AD by 60% [88]. These clinical benefits could be caused by direct effects of fish ω-3 PUFAs, EPA and DHA, on microglia and neurons, attenuating chronic neuroinflammation characterized by the pro-inflammatory and pro-apoptotic mediators associated with AD, PD, and ALS [89, 90]. Specific to microglia, ω-3 PUFAs have been shown to suppress inflammation by preventing harmful microglial activation, and by promoting the switch of activated microglia to an M2 protective phenotype [90].

Diverse types of antioxidants are present within the cells. A majority of non-enzymatic direct-acting antioxidants are derived from dietary sources [91]. Notable compounds in this class of antioxidants include vitamins C and E, β-carotene, coenzyme Q, and secondary plant metabolites such as polyphenols, nitrogen compounds and terpenoids [91]. Certain polyphenols in fruits, vegetables, and products manufactured from these groups such as wine, tea, and coffee, have been well characterized to have neuroprotective and anti-inflammatory activity in the CNS resulting from the disruption of chain oxidation reactions [92]. Murine microglial BV-2 cells pretreated with blueberry homogenate and subsequently stimulated with the endotoxin lipopolysaccharide (LPS) were shown to have significantly lowered cyclooxygenase (COX)-2 and iNOS expression, as well as decreased secretion of NO, IL-1β, and TNF-α [93]. Similar findings have been obtained by pretreating BV-2 cells with walnut and strawberry homogenates, as well as with polyphenolic-containing fractions of acai pulp [94]. The polyphenolic yellow curry spice curcumin has been shown to reduce microgliosis caused by intracerebroventricular infusion of Aβ in rats with efficacy similar to the non-steroidal anti-inflammatory drug ibuprofen [95]. Suppression of neuroinflammation by dietary curcumin could be a contributing factor to the observed ~75% lower incidence of AD in the Indian population in individuals over the age of 80 relative to the corresponding American population [95, 96].

According to 2012 data, caffeine-containing drinks constituted a $12.5 billion international market with over 80% of adult Americans consuming caffeine regularly [97, 98]. Consequently, several studies have aimed to determine the effects of caffeine on the neuropathologies of AD, PD, and ALS. Caffeine is an inhibitor of A_1 and A_{2A} adenosine receptors; blocking these receptors has been shown to reduce rat microglial activation and attenuate dopaminergic neurotoxicity in animal models of PD [99, 100]. Caffeine treatment was neuroprotective to dopaminergic neurons both prophylactically and when administered following the onset of the neurodegenerative process in rats exposed to the neurotoxin 1-methyl-4-phenylpyridinium [101]. Moreover, a study conducted with BV-2 cells concluded that caffeine was able to inhibit LPS-induced extracellular signal-regulated kinase (ERK) signaling, as well as Akt-dependent NF-κB activation, leading to decreased secretion of pro-inflammatory mediators NO, TNF-α, and PGE_2 [102]. Fiebich et al. [103] demonstrated that in addition to the inhibition of NF-κB activation, caffeine significantly reduced COX-2 protein synthesis in primary rat microglial cultures. Furthermore, a study conducted with a mouse PD model induced by 1-methyl-4-phenyl-1,2,3,6-tetrahydropyridine (MPTP) reported that caffeine suppressed the degradation of tight junction proteins occludin and ZO-1 by reducing transcription of metallomatrix protease 9, a tight junction protein-degrading enzyme [104]. Occludin and ZO-1 are critical proteins in maintaining the integrity of the BBB; its disruption has been implicated in the pathogenesis of several neurodegenerative disorders and as a central cause of AD; therefore, caffeine consumption has been suggested as a potential intervention in mitigating these disorders [104, 105]. Another potential means of reducing the prevalence of these diseases include staying active through regular physical activity.

3.2. Exercise

The health benefits of exercise have been well studied and it is universally understood that physical activity is crucial for maintaining a healthy body. Some of the well-known benefits of exercise include improved cardiovascular health and endurance, increased strength, enhanced metabolism, decreased adiposity (fat), as well as increased mood and mental health [106-110]. More recently, it has come to light that exercise has immune modifying capabilities, with an overall whole-body anti-inflammatory effect [106, 111-113]. Studies have revealed that physical activity 1) lowers numbers of circulating monocytes with the pro-inflammatory phenotype [106], 2) reduces levels of the circulating C-reactive protein (CRP) and the pro-inflammatory cytokines TNF-α and IL-1β, and 3) elevates levels of the anti-inflammatory cytokines IL-1 receptor antagonist (IL-1 RA) and IL-10 [111, 114-116]. Physical activity has also been shown to reduce the number of macrophages infiltrating between adipose cells in fatty tissue, and to switch the phenotype of adipose-embedded macrophages from a pro-inflammatory (M1) phenotype to an anti-inflammatory (M2) phenotype in obese rodents [117] and humans [118] alike. Research has shown that the systemic anti-inflammatory effect of exercise may be due to a reduction in density of toll-like receptors (TLR)-4, up to 50%, following bouts of acute as well as chronic training [106, 112, 119]. Downregulation of TLR-4 cell surface expression following exercise has been shown on monocytes, muscle, liver and adipose tissue [119, 120]. The mechanisms by which TLRs are downregulated following exercise is unknown.

Recently, inquiry into the beneficial effects of exercise has been extended to CNS processes and studies into the effects of physical activity on neuroinflammation have ensued. Kohman et al. [121] demonstrated that voluntary wheel running in aged mice attenuated microglia proliferation approximately 1.5 fold and reduced the number of M1 activated microglia approximately 1.8 fold. This study also established that voluntary exercise enhanced neurogenesis in aged mice by approximately 50%. Other studies have shown that voluntary exercise can be neuroprotective by reducing trimethyltin-induced neurotoxicity in the hippocampus of rodents [122]. This coincided with a reduction in the inflammatory markers IL-6, MCP-1 and TNF-α (approximately two-fold reduction for each). Rodent models of AD, which were introduced to moderate and intense physical activity, also showed a reduction in the number of activated microglia (up to 2.7 fold), as indicated by the microglia marker Iba-1 (ionized calcium binding adaptor molecule-1), and a reduction in the number of activated astrocytes (up to 9 fold), as indicated by the astrocytic marker glial fibrillary acidic protein (GFAP) [123]. This reduction in the number of activated glial cells correlated with a decline in the inflammatory markers COX-2, iNOS, TNF-α, IL-1β and IL-6 (approximately two fold each). These results are supported by similar studies using alternative mouse models of AD [124].

Long-term exercise can also reduce acute neuroinflammation caused by traumatic brain injury, as shown by a 1.4 fold decrease in lesion volume accompanied by a decrease in the pro-inflammatory cytokine IL-1β and an increase in the anti-inflammatory cytokine IL-10 in the brain [125]. This related to a 2.3 fold improvement in cognitive function, as defined by the standard Morris Water Maze test, in the exercise group compared to sedentary control mice.

To date, most studies regarding the anti-neuroinflammatory effect of exercise in the CNS have been performed in mice; however, some key research demonstrates that exercise reduces the probability of developing neurodegenerative diseases in humans, as well. Leading a sedentary lifestyle increases the risk of developing AD by up to 2.7 fold [10, 126], and PD by approximately two fold [127], while engaging in resistance training has shown to delay the progression of ALS as measured by the ALS Functional Rating Scale [128].

Exercise could be decreasing the incidence of several neurodegenerative diseases due to its anti-neuroinflammatory effects in the CNS. Although there are very few clinical studies in humans investigating exercise as a means of attenuating neuroinflammation, several experts propose that exercise could be a crucial therapeutic tool in reducing the incidence and severity of diseases that have a neuroinflammatory component [111, 123, 129-131]. Despite the wide range of beneficial effects of exercise, professional athletes involved in contact sports frequently experience head trauma, which is associated with increased risk for developing certain neurodegenerative diseases.

3.3. Head Injury

Traumatic brain injury (TBI) has been identified as one of the most consistently observed triggers for initiating the complex biochemical cascades that contribute to the pathology of AD, PD, and ALS [132-135]. TBI is defined as an external force to the head that exceeds the protective capacity of the brain thereby causing physical damage to the CNS, which leads to neurological impairments [136]. TBI may be described as mild, moderate, or severe, with 75% of injuries occurring as concussions or other mild TBIs repeatedly sustained by athletes in contact sports [137, 138]. As such, TBI is a highly heterogeneous disorder, etiology of which involves both primary and secondary injury mechanisms [137, 139]. The initial traumatic insult leads to mechanical damage of neurons, glial cells, and blood vessels caused by stretching, shearing, and/or tearing resulting in primary neuronal cell death [140]. Delayed cellular and metabolic changes triggered by the primary injury induce secondary injury, which exacerbates the initial damage and causes progressive neurodegeneration [141-145]. Chronic neuroinflammation is a well-established secondary injury mechanism in TBI and is also a common pathological feature of neurodegenerative disorders [139, 145]. Therefore, TBI has been implicated as a risk factor for AD, PD, and ALS, since prior TBI has been shown to increase the subsequent incidence of these neurodegenerative diseases [146].

Experimental and clinical research have identified neuroinflammation as a pathological response to brain injury. The role of non-neuronal glial cells in mediating such mechanisms of secondary TBI is becoming increasingly recognized [147-149]. Recently, activated microglia were found to be present in 28% of brains examined more than one year after a single TBI [150]. Post-mortem analysis of head injury survivors have also demonstrated increased microglial activation in the white matter up to 16 years after TBI [151]. Additional studies have revealed post-traumatic upregulation of microglial activation markers including CD68 and MHC-II [152]. Such findings point to the activation of resident microglia as a causative factor of neuroinflammation following TBI, which can have either beneficial and detrimental effects that differ in the acute and delayed phases after injury [139]. Upon induction of local brain injury *in vivo*, two-photon imaging of fluorescently labeled microglia showed rapid extension of ramified microglial processes towards the site of injury, which then fused to form a barrier between healthy and injured tissue [153]. The immediate chemotactic response of microglia caused by ATP released from the injured tissue is thought to contain the induced damage, thereby creating a stable environment for the restoration of functions in nearby neurons [153]. In addition, microglial activation in the acute phase of injury is accompanied by an increase in the secretion of anti-inflammatory cytokines such as IL-10 and transforming growth factor (TGF)-β, which are involved in neuronal protection and regeneration [143, 154, 155].

In contrast to the acute phase, the delayed phase in TBI is characterized by prolonged microglial activation observed in humans and animal models, which has been shown to have neurotoxic consequences [35, 156, 157]. Microglia express the TLR family of pattern recognition receptors (PRRs) capable of recognizing endogenously produced damage-associated molecular patterns (DAMPs) released by damaged cells [158, 159]. In addition, microglia have been found to express receptors for other factors secreted in excess following neuronal injury such as ATP and glutamate [160, 161]. Therefore, under the pathological conditions present following TBI, microglial cells could become chronically activated and mediate neuroinflammatory processes that trigger ongoing neuronal degeneration [162, 163]. Persistent activation of microglia is associated with increased secretion of pro-inflammatory cytokines such as IL-1β and TNF-α, which are elevated in the CSF of TBI patients and have been shown to mediate post-traumatic neuroinflammation with accompanying neuronal death [164-167]. Gene profiling studies in experimental models of TBI have demonstrated upregulated expression of other pro-inflammatory cytokines and chemokines characteristic of chronic microglial activation such as C-X-C motif chemokine (CXCL)-6, CXCL-10, IFN-γ, and IL-6 [152, 168, 169]. The influx of peripheral immune cells into the CNS has also been shown to occur in human TBI due to the disruption of the BBB following trauma to the brain, which results in the amplification of post-traumatic neuro-inflammation through the release of inflammatory molecules and further activation of microglial cells [170-172].

The neurotoxic effects of sustained microglial activation and chronic neuroinflammation have been demonstrated to contribute to the neurological dysfunction observed in TBI similar to other neurodegenerative disorders [139]. Recently, Mouzon et al. [173] showed that persistent neuroinflammation following repeated mild TBI in mice induced white matter degradation associated with long-term cognitive deficits. Similarly, Aungst et al. [174] demonstrated that repeated mild TBI in rats caused chronic microglial activation and neuroinflammation accompanied by hippocampal loss and cognitive impairments, which is similar to the changes observed in the brains of AD patients. In addition to the long-term damaging neuroinflammatory effects of TBI, other lifestyle associated factors contribute to the increased incidence of AD, PD and ALS. Once such category of lifestyle-associated risk factors includes diseases, which arise due to particular lifestyle choices.

3.4. Lifestyle-Associated Diseases and Conditions

Increasing incidences of lifestyle-related disorders, such as obesity, T2DM and metabolic syndrome, are plaguing the global population and putting tremendous stress on our health care systems. In addition to being classified as their own disorders, obesity, T2DM and metabolic syndrome are also well known risk factors for several other diseases and conditions [12, 175-177].

Obesity is defined as being grossly overweight, and is typically measured using the body mass index (BMI). The BMI is calculated based on weight and height, and having a BMI score of greater than 30 is considered to be a sign of obesity (Figure 4). According to the World Health Organization, today more than 1.9 billion adults (over the age of 18) are obese, while 600 million children (under the age of 18) are obese worldwide [178]. Obesity has recently been classified as a disease state, and is a risk factor for several other peripheral disorders such as T2DM, and cardiovascular disease [179]. High BMI and midlife obesity increase the risk of developing AD approximately two fold [11] and obese women have been shown to have an onset of AD on average four years earlier than their non-obese counterparts [175, 180]. Other studies have shown that obesity increases the risk of developing PD by up to 74%, compared to normal weight individuals [12, 181].

Contrary to the findings that high BMI contributes to an increased risk for AD and PD, research suggests that low BMI is associated with developing ALS, showing that BMI of less than 18 (under-weight), correlated with a 1.6 RR of developing ALS [10, 182]. However, the latter finding for ALS may not be due to a cause and effect relationship, but rather may indicate that the hypermetabolic state in ALS precedes the onset of the detectable clinical disease by many years [183].

T2DM is a metabolic disorder characterized by hyperglycemia caused by functional insulin resistance. T2DM is a growing epidemic, currently affecting upwards of 347 million people worldwide, and the prevalence of T2DM is on the rise [184]. This is especially alarming, since T2DM has been identified as a risk factor for developing additional diseases such as AD, PD, ALS and cardiovascular disease [179, 185, 186]. Therefore, as the incidence of T2DM increases, it is inevitable that the incidence of AD, PD and ALS will also increase.

Body Mass Index (BMI)		
Calculation	**BMI Score**	**Weight Category**
$BMI = \dfrac{Weight\ (lbs)\ x\ 703}{Height\ (in)^2}$	< 18.5	Underweight
	18.5 – 25	Normal Weight
OR	25 – 30	Overweight
$BMI = \dfrac{Weight\ (kg)}{Height\ (m)^2}$	30 – 40	Obese
	> 40	Morbidly Obese

Figure 4. Body Mass Index (BMI) calculations and weight categories according to BMI score.

Metabolic syndrome, formerly known as syndrome X, is a newly defined condition, characterized by hypertension, hyperglycemia, hypertriglyceride-mia, reduced high-density lipoprotein cholesterol and abdominal obesity, which is often accompanied by other symptoms such as chest pains or shortness of breath, neuropathy and retinopathy [177]. Metabolic syndrome is a manifestation of potentially very serious clinical condition, which also contributes to the incidence of AD and PD [187-189], while research regarding the relationship between metabolic syndrome and ALS is limited.

Studies have shown that obesity is a risk factor for developing AD, with a RR of up to 1.80, and that T2DM is associated with a RR of approximately 1.54 for developing AD [126]. Studies have also shown that AD patients with metabolic syndrome have significantly lower scores on the Mini Mental State Examination for cognitive impairment (on average 9% lower score) compared to AD patients who do not have metabolic syndrome [176].

Similar to the findings for AD, obesity, T2DM and metabolic syndrome have all been identified as significant risk factors for PD [189]. Mid-life obesity has been shown to enhance the risk of developing PD by 74%, and being overweight increases the risk of developing PD by 34% [181], while an additional study showed that morbid obesity can increase the risk of PD by a RR of up to 2.44 [190]. Other studies have shown that T2DM increases the RR of developing PD by a factor of 1.8 [185]. The combined risk factors for PD, including hypertension, obesity and insulin resistance point to metabolic syndrome as being an important and growing risk factor for this neurodegenerative disease [189]. Very little research has been conducted on the relationship between T2DM and ALS; however, a study by Jawaid et al. [191] suggested that patients with T2DM and ALS present with a delayed onset of motor symptoms, compared to the ALS patients without T2DM.

One of the common features of the three main lifestyle-associated conditions is the state of chronic peripheral inflammation. High levels of adiposity, found in obesity, metabolic syndrome and typically T2DM, are associated with a chronic systemic inflammatory environment and elevated levels of circulating inflammatory cytokines such as IL-6, IL-1β and TNF-α [130, 192, 193]. This may be due, in part, to the increased infiltration of macrophages into adipose tissue, and a switch in their phenotype from M2 to M1 [194]. Other common examples of inflammation in these three conditions include increased circulating levels of CRP and decreased endothelial function [111, 195, 196]. This is important to note, since the decrease in function of the endothelial cells could lead to a leaky BBB, resulting in the increased passage of cytokines and inflammatory mediators from the periphery into the CNS [130, 197]. Animal studies have shown that obese mice exhibit increased infiltration of macrophages from the periphery into the CNS, by up to 53% above the controls [198]. Moreover, since inflammatory molecules such as MCP-1 regulate tight junctions at the BBB [199], this increased infiltration may be due to the chronic state of peripheral inflammation.

It is possible that peripheral inflammation linked to lifestyle-associated conditions has the potential to initiate or propagate an environment of neuroinflammation. Several studies have demonstrated that obese rodents have elevated markers of neuroinflammation including increased levels of the pro-inflammatory cytokines IL-6 and TNF-α (approximate 1.5 fold increase in the hippocampus), as well as increased activity of NF-κB, enhanced infiltration of peripheral immune cells and activation of microglia within the CNS [200, 201]. This may be due to the increased deterioration of the BBB, which is associated with obesity, and would allow for the free passage of cytokines and peripheral immune cells across the BBB [202].

Diabetic rats have repeatedly shown cognitive impairment accompanied by elevated levels of inflammatory cytokines. These experiments have shown that diabetic rodents exhibit enhanced neuroinflammation, up to a two fold increase in IL-1β and TNF-α and a 1.5 fold increase in microgliosis (indicated by the microglia marker Iba-1). Administration of the anti-diabetic drugs metformin or liraglutide reduces cognitive deficits and neuroinflammation to non-diabetic levels [203, 204].

While to date only few studies have looked specifically at the contribution of metabolic syndrome to neuroinflammation, several studies have investigated individual aspects of metabolic syndrome as potential contributing factors for neuroinflammation. In addition to the previously discussed risk factors for neuroinflammation (obesity and T2DM) several other metabolic syndrome complications have been identified as potential inducers of neuroinflammation. For example, dyslipidemia is characterized by the release of surplus free fatty acids. When fatty acids cross the BBB in excess, they can induce pro-inflammatory effects, such as enhanced cytokine secretion (MCP-1, IL-6 and TNF-α) by glial cells, and glia-mediated neurotoxicity [205, 206]. Furthermore, hyperglycemia, a hallmark of metabolic syndrome, can lead to the formation of advanced glycation end products (AGEs), which are glycated proteins that typically suffer a reduction in protein function. AGEs have been shown to be very destructive to endothelial tissues and to be able to degrade the BBB [207], which could allow for peripheral inflammation associated with metabolic syndrome to transcend the BBB and create an environment of neuroinflammation. Therefore, the common underlying feature linking obesity, T2DM and metabolic syndrome with a risk for developing AD, PD and ALS may be the chronic inflammatory environment.

3.5. Substance Abuse

3.5.1. Alcohol

The chronic inflammatory environment present in AD, PD and ALS brain can be attenuated or exacerbated through the use of alcohol and certain drugs (Figure 5). Alcohol has been utilized by humans for thousands of years and is one of the most consumed drugs in present day. Alcohol has been used as a euphoriant to accompany positive social and religious occasions [208]. However, serious adverse effects caused by chronic use or abuse of alcohol have been recognized over the past few decades [209]. In addition to the well-established social corollaries, such as becoming ostracized from family or friends, alcohol abuse could lead to serious physical consequences, such as cirrhosis of the liver and facilitation of neuroinflammation in the brain which, as mentioned previously, is a hallmark shared by AD, PD and ALS [208, 210].

Chronic alcohol use is associated with a decrease in immune system function accompanied by increased levels of pro-inflammatory cytokines and chemokines [211]. A review by Crews et al. [212] illustrated that long-term alcohol use triggered neuroinflammatory processes involving TNF-α, IL-1β and MCP-1 released by activated glial cells. Pascual et al. [213] confirmed these observations through the use of animal models. They demonstrated that chronic alcohol exposure in mice increased the brain levels of the pro-inflammatory cytokines IL-17, IL-1β and TNF-α, as well as the chemokines MCP-1, macrophage inflammatory protein-1a (MIP-1a) and fractalkine (CX_3CL1) by up to two fold [213].

Recently, TNF-α has become regarded as one of the most significant pro-inflammatory cytokines involved in alcohol-induced neuroinflammation. Studies have shown that TNF-α, once released, plays an important role by inducing the secretion of other cytokines involved in pro-inflammatory processes; therefore, TNF-α could be the key molecule exacerbating the effects of alcohol in the development of neurodegenerative diseases including AD, PD and ALS [214].

The relationship between alcohol consumption and neuroinflammation is not as one-sided as it may seem, however. Novel research has indicated that pre-existing neuroinflammation may promote the consumption of alcohol and contribute to the development of alcohol dependence [215]. Excessive alcohol use and abuse has been linked with abnormalities in both cognitive and motor function, as well as deficits in impulse and behavioral control, which could contribute to further consumption of alcohol, and therefore further promote neuroinflammation and the progression of neurodegenerative diseases [214]. Bajo et al. [215] identified the central amygdala as a significant contributor to the development of alcohol dependence. Initial research on this topic showed that chronic alcohol exposure led to a decrease in transmission of gamma-aminobutyric acid (GABA), the main inhibitory neurotransmitter of the brain. This reduction in GABAergic transmission, both pre- and post-synaptically, was associated with the development of alcohol dependence and increased alcohol consumption [216]. Bajo et al. [215], however, demonstrated that increasing levels of IL-1β increased GABAergic transmission in some brain areas, such as the hypothalamus and hippocampus, while decreasing GABAergic transmission in other brain areas such as the cerebellum and basolateral amygdala. The results of this study indicated that variance in GABAergic transmission could be brain region specific and contribute to the complex interactions involved in the development of alcohol dependence [215].

Overall, long-term alcohol consumption could have varying aversive physiological effects. Some of the associated repercussions include microgliosis accompanied by increased levels of pro-inflammatory cytokines, which can lead to irreversible brain damage [213], neuroinflammation and the development of neurodegenerative diseases including AD and PD [217, 218].

3.5.2. Nicotine

Nicotine, on the other hand, is associated with having anti-inflammatory properties. Nicotine produces its anti-inflammatory effects by selectively targeting the α7 nicotinic acetylcholine receptor (α7nAChR), which plays a critical role in maintaining homeostatic inflammatory responses throughout the body and brain [219]. One of the ways the α7nAChR regulates inflammation is through the cholinergic anti-inflammatory pathway. This pathway helps to ensure that the inflammatory response is balanced to prevent cell damage and death from occurring [220]. The α7nAChR, which is expressed on microglia throughout the CNS and on macrophages of the peripheral immune system, becomes activated in the presence of nicotine, acetylcholine, or one of their derivatives [219-221]. Activation of this receptor inhibits the production of pro-inflammatory cytokines, including TNF-α, IL-1β and IL-6, while the production of anti-inflammatory cytokines, including IL-10, remains unaffected [222]. These anti-inflammatory effects occur in both the peripheral and central nervous systems. Recent analysis has demonstrated that nicotine, along with some of its derivatives, reduces neuroinflammation and promotes synaptic plasticity in neurons [219, 221]. By using animal models, it was confirmed that activation of the α7nAChR generated an anti-inflammatory effect that led to the promotion of neuron survival, especially in the brain regions most significantly affected by PD pathology [219, 223].

Over the past few decades, the aversive effects of tobacco smoking, the most popular route of administration for nicotine, have become very evident. Nicotine has become regarded as extremely addictive [224], and chronic use or abuse of tobacco has been identified as a risk factor in the development of many disorders, including lung cancer [225], coronary heart disease [226] and chronic obstructive pulmonary disease [227]. Despite the many aversive effects of long-term tobacco use, it has been suggested that nicotine, as well as some of its derivatives, has anti-inflammatory properties that could reduce neuroinflammation and assist in the treatment of various maladies including PD [218, 219]. Future studies may be necessary to determine the safest route of administration of nicotine, as the risks currently associated with tobacco smoke far outweigh the possible benefits of nicotine.

3.5.3. Psychostimulant Drugs

Psychostimulant drugs, including cocaine and amphetamines, have been used medicinally. It was not until recently, however, that the recreational uses for these drugs gained popularity. Cocaine and amphetamines, including methamphetamine (Meth) and 3,4-methlenedioxymethamphetamine (MDMA or "ecstasy"), produce a sense of euphoria accompanied by heightened attention and decreased fatigue [208]. These effects allow the user to reduce stress and become more efficient during work- or school-related tasks [228].

Recent studies have determined that the presence of cocaine, Meth and MDMA within the CNS have profound effects on the functioning and regulation of important immune-related cell signaling pathways [228-230]. Chronic use and abuse of these substances is associated with increased astrocyte activation, as indicated by an increase in the expression of the astrogliosis marker GFAP, and upregulated production of pro-inflammatory cytokines including TNF-α, IL-1β, IFN-γ, and MCP-1, creating an inflammatory environment, which contributes to neuronal death and subsequent development of neurodegenerative diseases [228, 231, 232]. In addition, cocaine use is associated with the upregulation of additional cytokines, including IL-6, which are involved in altering the expression of tight junction proteins and increasing the activation of BBB remodeling enzymes [229]. This, in turn, increases the permeability of the BBB and decreases its functionality, therefore allowing peripheral inflammatory mediators and neurotoxic compounds to cross into the CNS. This disruption and infiltration of the BBB can result in neuroinflammation and neuronal damage [230, 233], which could increase the susceptibility of an individual to develop neurodegenerative disorders including AD, PD and ALS [228, 229, 232].

3.5.4. Opiates

Opiates, including morphine and heroin, have been utilized for many decades due to their powerful analgesic effects. In the 1970s, many researchers were interested in the mechanism of action of this class of drug. This led to the discovery of a class of brain chemicals, called endorphins, which act in the body as the endogenous pain-relieving system [208, 234]. More recent studies have demonstrated that opiate drugs, due to their similarity in structure to endorphins, are able to bind to and activate the endorphin system of the brain, thereby producing analgesic effects. Serious physical and social consequences are also associated with chronic use and abuse of opiates, however, as they are extremely addictive [208].

Recent research has revealed that opiates possess immunomodulatory properties that may play a significant role in both neuroinflammation and neurodegenerative diseases. Morphine, a naturally occurring opiate, exerts its CNS effects by acting on three classes of opioid receptors (μ, δ and κ) to upregulate the production of MCP-1, which plays a significant role in the recruitment of monocytes/macrophages, neutrophils and lymphocytes to impaired areas within the brain [235, 236].

Heroin, a synthetic opiate, is considered to be twice as potent as morphine, as it crosses the BBB more readily [208]. Heroin, like morphine, has immunomodulatory properties that can induce neuroinflammatory response. Recent studies have demonstrated that the presence of heroin in the CNS induces the production and release of pro-inflammatory cytokines TNF-α, IL-1β, and IL-6 [237]. Therefore, it is evident that chronic use and abuse of opiates can lead to the overproduction of pro-inflammatory cytokines and immune cells, which can play a significant role in neuroinflammatory response and the development and progression of neurodegenerative diseases including AD, PD and ALS.

3.5.5. Antidepressants

Relatively high occurrence of depression (major depressive disorder, MDD) has been noted amongst individuals afflicted with neurodegenerative disease (discussed in section 3.6) [238, 239]. Depression is another multifaceted disease in which inflammatory pathways may be chronically active [240]. MDD is primarily characterized by an imbalance in several of the key monoamine neurotransmitters of the brain, such as norepinephrine (noradrenaline), serotonin (5-HT), dopamine and epinephrine (adrenaline). These neurotransmitters not only control neurons, but can also modulate the neuroimmune status of the CNS including regulation of glial cell functions; therefore, their dysregulated secretion can have pathological outcomes. Norepinephrine is thought to have an immunosuppressive role in a healthy brain, and thus it is not surprising that in AD and PD pathology, the reduction of noradrenergic signaling can cause hyperactivation of the immune system [241]. Decreased 5-HT signaling is implicated in reduced cognitive ability in AD [242]. In contrast, in ALS both norepinephrine and 5-HT can exacerbate the motor neuron hyperexcitability prevalent in this pathology [239]. Currently, common therapies for the treatment of depression are directed at modulating the monoaminergic pathways with the main goal of increasing intrasynaptic monoamine neurotransmitters [243]. The ability of monoamine neurotransmitters to be neuroprotective or immunosuppressive implies a potential utility of antidepressants in AD and PD treatment. There are several different classes of antidepressants, including tricyclic antidepressants (TCA), serotonin/norepinephrine reuptake inhibitors (SNRI), serotonin selective reuptake inhibitors (SSRI), monoamine oxidase inhibitors (MAOIs), atypical receptor blocking compounds and new therapies such as *N*-methyl-D-aspartate (NMDA) receptor antagonists. The different classes of antidepressants will be discussed with regards to their potential effects on neurodegeneration and neuroinflammation.

TCAs are thought to operate by competitively blocking the pre-synaptic reuptake of norepinephrine and 5-HT [243]. As reuptake is blocked, the availability of monoamines both transmitted within the synaptic cleft and received by the post-synaptic neuron is increased. Imipramine is a TCA with some anti-inflammatory effects related to decreased NF-κB signaling, as well as lowered expression of iNOS, IL-1β, and TNF-α, as demonstrated in murine microglial cells [244]. In primary rat astrocytes, imipramine decreased nuclear translocation of NF-κB, which is required for cellular signaling and release of pro-inflammatory cytokines [245]. However, use of imipramine and other TCAs is associated with high risk of adverse effects such as hepatotoxicity, and high mortality with overdose [243, 246].

SSRIs block the pre-synaptic reuptake of 5-HT, and similarly SNRIs non-selectively block pre-synaptic 5-HT and norepinephrine reuptake. Adjunctive medications are often required for SSRIs and SNRIs in treating MDD due to the low efficacy of SSRIs/SNRIs alone [238]. As suggested by a meta-analysis, however, SSRIs may be more effective at reducing levels of circulating pro-inflammatory cytokines; although caution must be exercised as there are few thorough studies of this anti-inflammatory effect [247].

Pro-inflammatory effects of SSRIs have also been detected; thus, sertraline (an SSRI) increased pro-inflammatory IL-6 expression in human hippocampal progenitor cells [248]. Another study found sertraline to exhibit anti-inflammatory effects with decreased levels of NO and TNF-α at high sertraline concentrations in microglial cell culture [249]. Such inconsistent results may stem from the heterogeneity in dosage regimens between different experiments. Results such as these seem common for antidepressant effects related to neuroinflammation, and are similar for other SSRIs, such as fluoxetine [250]. For example, it has been reported that fluoxetine had no impact on disease progression in the ALS murine model, although its effects on neuroinflammation were not specifically studied [239].

Few studies of antidepressants detail their pro-inflammatory effect. For example, an increase in IL-1β mRNA was found in the hypothalamus following administration of the SNRI desipramine to rats [251]. Of note, IL-1 receptor type 2 was also upregulated, which is a decoy receptor that helps regulate levels of IL-1β [252]; therefore, this increase of IL-1β may not have been long-lived. Another study described the anti-inflammatory action of desipramine (an SNRI), which inhibited expression of pro-inflammatory chemokines and cell adhesion molecules in rat cortex [241]. Venlafaxine is an SNRI with a preference for the 5-HT reuptake transporter, which also inhibits the norepinephrine reuptake [238, 253]. In 2002 it was considered to be one of the best treatment options of MDD [253]. While some research describes little to no anti-inflammatory activity of venlafaxine, other studies have demonstrated an anti-inflammatory effect in human hippocampal progenitor cells [248, 249]. Thus, while SSRIs and SNRIs may provide a basis for treatment of neuroinflammation, care must be taken to not over-interpret the utility of these drugs, as further studies are needed to elucidate their effectiveness as anti-inflammatory agents.

MAOIs operate by reversibly or irreversibly binding to the enzyme monoamine oxidase; this enzyme breaks down monoamine neurotransmitters, producing H_2O_2 and ROS, and thus is associated with PD pathology [254]. The monoamine oxidase (MAO)-A form is usually responsible for the breakdown of neurotransmitters norepinephrine, 5-HT and epinephrine [255]. The MAO-B form typically breaks down dopamine and β-phenylethylamine. Ladostigil is a MAO-B inhibitor that was shown to reduce iNOS expression, along with IL-1β, IL-6, and TNF-α expression in rat parietal cortex to levels similar to that of the younger control group [256]. High levels of these mediators were suggested to be age-related in this rat model. Reduction in IL-1β, IL-6 and TNF-α by ladostigil was replicated in LPS-activated murine microglial cultures. These anti-inflammatory effects were found to be separate from the MAO inhibitory activity of ladostigil. In addition, ladostigil at clinically-relevant concentrations was shown to slow down age-related deterioration in spatial memory [256].

Rasagiline is a MAO-B inhibitor and is a current treatment option for PD [257]. Interestingly, the utility of MAO inhibitors in PD is thought to stem from their irreversible MAO-B inhibitory properties as well as additional anti-inflammatory activity [257]. Rasagiline was shown to reduce IL-6 and IL-1β levels, as well as ROS and NO levels in microglial cultures prepared from DJ-

1 deficient mice, which mimic a form of PD with a single gene deficiency [254]. The inhibition of ROS and NO was suggested to be dependent on the MAO inhibition by rasagiline [254].

In contrast to the TCAs, SSRIs, SNRIs and MAOIs, which act to increase levels of monoamine neurotransmitters in the synaptic cleft of neurons, NMDA receptor antagonists have a distinct mode of action. Glutamate binds to the NMDA receptor, and is known to elicit excitatory functions in the brain [258]. When this function is altered, deterioration of neuroplasticity can occur [238]. Dysregulation of glutamate transmission is implicated in PD pathology [259]. Furthermore, over-activation of NMDA receptors located outside of the synapse has been linked to the pathogenesis of AD [260]. In ALS, the current therapeutic riluzole operates by disrupting glutamate release with the aim of reducing motor neuron excitability, pathologically related to the disease state of ALS [239]. Ketamine, a NMDA receptor antagonist, has an established high efficacy in treating MDD, though it carries safety concerns as it is administered intravenously and has the potential to be addictive [258]. Although the effect of ketamine on neuroinflammation has not been fully elucidated, it may act in a regulatory manner, having potential pro- and anti-inflammatory effects [261]. Ketamine elicited IL-6 and TNF-α upregulation in a monocyte/macrophage cell culture, independent of the blockage of NMDA receptor function [261]. In contrast, ketamine was also responsible for reducing levels of NO, TNF-α and IL-1β as well as nuclear translocation of NF-κB in another macrophage cell culture [262]. The diversity of effects lend support to the suggested regulatory role of ketamine. NMDA receptor antagonists such as ketamine have the potential to be a very innovative treatment for a multitude of diseases, and as such more research is required to determine their safety and efficacy related to CNS diseases and depression.

This brief review of interactions between current antidepressant therapies and neuroinflammation illustrates the potential for this class of drugs in treatment of neurodegenerative diseases. Further studies will be required to elucidate the precise effects of antidepressants on neuroinflammation, perhaps specifically in areas most affected by the neurodegenerative disorders, such as the substantia nigra in PD, the hippocampus in AD, and the motor cortex in ALS [254, 263, 264].

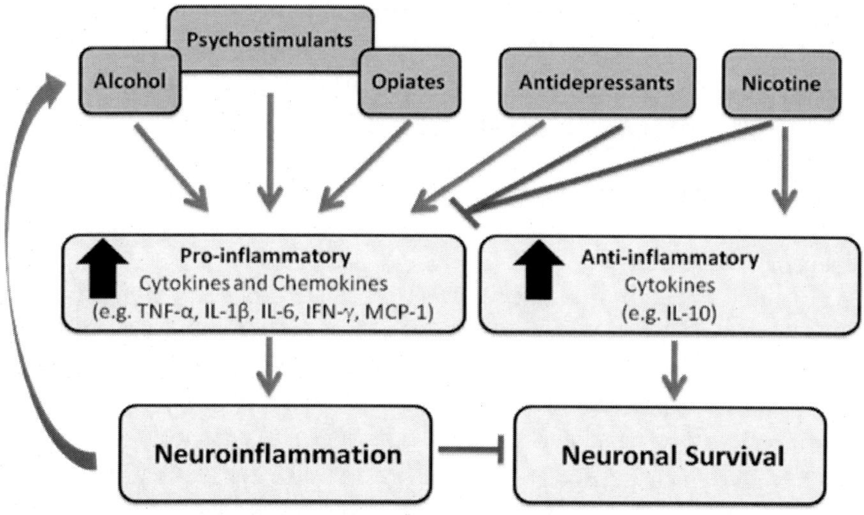

Figure 5. Substance abuse can have immunomodulatory effects in the CNS, resulting in enhanced neuronal survival or neuroinflammation accompanied by neurodegeneration.

3.6. Psychological and Emotional Health

Stress and MDD are associated with an increased risk of developing AD and could also lead to neuroinflammation [265-268]. The psychological and emotional health of an individual affects the production of pro-inflammatory cytokines, including TNF-α and IFN-γ [266, 268]. Activation of the CNS immune system by these cytokines results in the upregulation of indoleamine 2,3-dioxygenase (IDO) and corticotropin-releasing hormone (CRH), which perpetuate the neuroinflammation cascade induced by depression and stress [269, 270].

Individuals afflicted with AD have shown high comorbidity with depression. As such, MDD is one of the earliest neuropsychiatric abnormalities to develop in AD patients [271, 272]. It is possible that the high comorbidity between AD and MDD is due to a number of shared pro-inflammatory factors such as IL-1β, TNF-α and pro-apoptotic markers [272]. Elevated pro-inflammatory cytokine levels have been found in the plasma and CSF of patients with depression, showing activation of their immune system [266]. Using stress-induction in animal models, Liu et al. [273] demonstrated that depression correlated with an increase in the pro-inflammatory cytokines TNF-α and IFN-γ in the prefrontal cortex. Pro-inflammatory cytokines exacerbated neurodegeneration as seen by the atrophy of the hippocampus and frontal cortex brain regions that are linked to both depression and AD [269]. Depression can also be an early symptom of neurodegeneration as concluded by a 14 year study of healthy patients, who first developed MDD, followed by AD later on in life [267]. The correlation between MDD and AD has been well documented and further research has been directed at characterizing the mechanistic connections between the psychological illness and the neuro-degenerative disease.

The link between AD and MDD is speculated to result from systemic inflammation, which plays an important role in protecting an organism and promoting recovery. Systemic infection leads to behaviors commonly referred to as "sickness behaviors," which include depression [270]. Injections of LPS into mice led to exaggerated sickness behaviors and enhanced synthesis of IDO mRNA, which is associated with depressive-like behaviors [270]. There is evidence that IDO, a ubiquitously expressed enzyme, has a prominent role in triggering chronic inflammation within the CNS, as well as in the development of LPS- and pro-inflammatory cytokine-induced MDD [274]. Quinolinic acid, the end product of the catabolic tryptophan pathway triggered by IDO is a neurotoxic activator of the NMDA receptor, which contributes to excitotoxicity in neurodegenerative disease [274]. O'Connor et al. [275] revealed that IFN-γ and TNF-α synergistically induce IDO expression in primary murine microglia inoculated with the bacterium bacilli Calmette-Guérin. Activation of IDO by pro-inflammatory cytokines led to the generation of several neuroactive metabolites, including quinolinic acid, which are implicated in neurodegenerative disorders [275].

In addition to being recognized as a hallmark of neurodegenerative diseases, neuroinflammation is now known to be an important biological event that increases the occurrence of major depressive episodes [276]. Psychosocial stress can activate the inflammatory response both in the periphery and the CNS; therefore, stress may be linked to depression through inflammation [266, 277]. Recent evidence has revealed that TNF-α mRNA levels are significantly upregulated in mice subjected to stress, demonstrating the role of stress in the development of neuroinflammation [268]. Chronic unpredictable mild stress (CUMS) induced by unfavorable living conditions increased the levels of pro-inflammatory cytokines TNF-α and IFN-γ in the prefrontal cortex of mice [273]. Stress exposure also increased inflammatory gene transcription and stimulated astrogliosis, which play a significant role in the neuroinflammation response characteristic of AD [268]. By surveying 1,064 people, it was shown that self-reported stress (distress proneness) is a risk factor for developing AD

[265]. Stress-induced hormone release has been shown to be a biochemical risk factor for neurodegenerative disorders.

The hypothalamus–pituitary–adrenal (HPA) axis is a neuroendocrine system that induces the production of cortisol, a stress hormone released by the adrenal glands [278]. CRH, which is also released in response to stress, is the main brain peptide involved in the activation of the HPA axis [278]. Within the HPA axis, cortisol mediates the negative feedback on CRH secretion by binding to the cortisol receptors located in the hypothalamus and hippocampus. CRH has a wide variety of activities that are mediated by two distinct G-protein-coupled receptors, corticotropin releasing hormone receptors (CRH-R) 1 and 2, which have different expression patterns in the brain [279]. CRH is also associated with activation of an immune response that results in increased release of pro-inflammatory cytokines. In turn, pro-inflammatory cytokines activate the HPA axis leading to further release of CRH, as well as reduced sensitivity to glucocorticoid hormone, thereby impairing the regulatory feedback mechanism and exacerbating pro-inflammatory cytokine release [269]. It can be seen through the regulation of the HPA axis by CRH that stress can be a risk factor for neuroinflammation and consequently neurodegenerative diseases including AD, PD and ALS.

Conclusion

AD, PD and ALS are prevalent neurodegenerative diseases that share neuroinflammation as a common underlying mechanism contributing to the disease progression. Dysregulated microglial activation in these diseases, if prolonged, can result in microgliosis, which is accompanied by the increased and sustained release of pro-inflammatory mediators. Due to its non-specific nature, the pro-inflammatory response can result in collateral damage to the surrounding neurons and may contribute to the neurodegeneration observed in AD, PD and ALS.

Over the years, several non-modifiable risk factors for developing AD, PD and ALS have been identified, including genetic components and exposure to environmental neurotoxins. This knowledge has helped to elucidate the mechanisms involved in disease onset and progression. The discovery of modifiable risk factors that can facilitate and modify the neuroinflammatory environment found in AD, PD and ALS has allowed for the development of novel therapeutic and lifestyle interventions, in addition to the more classic drug-based therapies. Studies on the role of diet, exercise, as well as psychological and emotional health have demonstrated that these modifiable risk factors are of great importance for understanding the pathology of neurodegenerative diseases. Furthermore, by introducing lifestyle changes, such as increasing physical activity and reducing stress levels, both individual risk and overall prevalence of these diseases can be significantly reduced.

Overall, controlling the modifiable risk factors could be a more effective strategy for reducing neuroinflammation than trying to inhibit or reverse the already established inflammatory environment. Preventing the progression from acute to chronic inflammation in the CNS may help more effectively to decrease the risk of developing neurodegenerative diseases such as AD, PD and ALS.

Acknowledgments

This work was supported by grants from the Jack Brown and Family Alzheimer's Disease Research Foundation, the Natural Science and Engineering Research Council of Canada and the University of British Columbia Okanagan Campus.

References

[1]   Alzheimer's Disease International (2009). *World Alzheimer Report Executive Summary*. [cited June 08,2015].

[2]   Parkinson's Disease Foundation (2010). *Understanding Parkinson's- Parkinson's FAQ*. [cited June 08,2015].

[3]   The International Alliance of ALS/MND Associations (2015). *The International Alliance of ALS/MND Associations*. [cited June 08,2015].

[4]   Daviglus, M. L., Bell, C. C., Berrettini, W., Bowen, P. E., Connolly, E. S., Jr., Cox, N. J., Dunbar-Jacob, J. M., et al. (2010). National Institutes of Health State-of-the-Science Conference statement: preventing alzheimer disease and cognitive decline. *Ann Intern Med, 153*, 176-181.

[5]   Adams, H. H., de Bruijn, R. F., Hofman, A., Uitterlinden, A. G., van Duijn, C. M., Vernooij, M. W., Koudstaal, P. J., et al. (2015). Genetic risk of neurodegenerative diseases is associated with mild cognitive impairment and conversion to dementia. *Alzheimers Dement, 15*, 1-9.

[6]   Chen, S., Sayana, P., Zhang, X. & Le, W. (2013). Genetics of amyotrophic lateral sclerosis: an update. *Mol Neurodegener*, *8*, 1-15.

[7]   Trudler, D., Nash, Y. & Frenkel, D. (2015). New insights on Parkinson's disease genes: the link between mitochondria impairment and neuroinflammation. *J Neural Transm*, *1355*, 1-11.

[8]   Chin-Chan, M., Navarro-Yepes, J. & Quintanilla-Vega, B. (2015). Environmental pollutants as risk factors for neurodegenerative disorders: Alzheimer and Parkinson diseases. *Front Cell Neurosci*, *9*, 124.

[9]   Jomova, K., Vondrakova, D., Lawson, M. & Valko, M. (2010). Metals, oxidative stress and neurodegenerative disorders. *Mol Cell Biochem*, *345*, 91-104.

[10]   Scarmeas, N., Luchsinger, J. A., Schupf, N., Brickman, A. M., Cosentino, S., Tang, M. X. & Stern, Y. (2009). Physical activity, diet, and risk of Alzheimer disease. *JAMA*, *302*, 627-637.

[11]   Whitmer, R. A., Gunderson, E. P., Quesenberry, C. P., Jr., Zhou, J. & Yaffe, K. (2007). Body mass index in midlife and risk of Alzheimer disease and vascular dementia. *Curr Alzheimer Res*, *4*, 103-109.

[12]   Chen, J., Guan, Z., Wang, L., Song, G., Ma, B. & Wang, Y. (2014). Meta-analysis: overweight, obesity, and Parkinson's disease. *Int J Endocrinol*, *2014*, 203930.

[13]   Lambert, J. C., Ibrahim-Verbaas, C. A., Harold, D., Naj, A. C., Sims, R., Bellenguez, C., DeStafano, A. L., et al. (2013). Meta-analysis of 74,046 individuals identifies 11 new susceptibility loci for Alzheimer's disease. *Nat Genet*, *45*, 1452-1458.

[14]   Lill, C. M., Roehr, J. T., McQueen, M. B., Kavvoura, F. K., Bagade, S., Schjeide, B. M., Schjeide, L. M., et al. (2012). Comprehensive research synopsis and systematic meta-analyses in Parkinson's disease genetics: The PDGene database. *PLoS Genet*, *8*, e1002548.

[15]   Plagnol V, Nalls M.A., B. J. M., Hernandez D.G., Sharma M., Sheerin U.M., Saad M., Simón-Sánchez J., et al. (2011). A two-stage meta-analysis identifies several new loci for Parkinson's disease. *PLoS Genet*, *7*, e1002142.

[16]   Fogh, I., Ratti, A., Gellera, C., Lin, K., Tiloca, C., Moskvina, V., Corrado, L., et al. (2014). A genome-wide association meta-analysis identifies a novel locus at 17q11.2 associated with sporadic amyotrophic lateral sclerosis. *Hum Mol Genet*, *23*, 2220-2231.

[17]   Goate, A., Chartier-Harlin, M. C., Mullan, M., Brown, J., Crawford, F., Fidani, L., Giuffra, L., et al. (1991). Segregation of a missense mutation

in the amyloid precursor protein gene with familial Alzheimer's disease. *Nature, 349*, 704-706.

[18] Tang, Y.-P. & Gershon, E. S. (2003). Genetic studies in Alzheimer's disease. *Dialogues Clin Neurosci, 5*, 17-26.

[19] Li, J. Q., Tan, L., Wang, H. F., Tan, M. S., Xu, W., Zhao, Q. F., Wang, J., et al. (2015). Risk factors for predicting progression from mild cognitive impairment to Alzheimer's disease: a systematic review and meta-analysis of cohort studies. *J Neurol Neurosurg Psychiatry, 2014*, 1-9.

[20] Miller, D. W., Hague, S. M., Clarimon, J., Baptista, M., Gwinn-Hardy, K., Cookson, M. R. & Singleton, A. B. (2004). Alpha-synuclein in blood and brain from familial Parkinson disease with SNCA locus triplication. *Neurology, 62*, 1835-1838.

[21] Singleton, A. B., Farrer, M., Johnson, J., Singleton, A., Hague, S., Kachergus, J., Hulihan, M., et al. (2003). alpha-Synuclein locus triplication causes Parkinson's disease. *Science, 302*, 841.

[22] Cheon, S. M., Chan, L., Chan, D. K. & Kim, J. W. (2012). Genetics of Parkinson's disease - a clinical perspective. *J Mov Disord, 5*, 33-41.

[23] Paez-Colasante, X., Figueroa-Romero, C., Sakowski, S. A., Goutman, S. A. & Feldman, E. L. (2015). Amyotrophic lateral sclerosis: mechanisms and therapeutics in the epigenomic era. *Nat Rev Neurol*, 1-14.

[24] Ingre, C., Roos, P. M., Piehl, F., Kamel, F. & Fang, F. (2015). Risk factors for amyotrophic lateral sclerosis. *Clin Epidemiol, 7*, 181-193.

[25] Park, J. H., Lee, D. W., Park, K. S. & Joung, H. (2014). Serum trace metal levels in Alzheimer's disease and normal control groups. *Am J Alzheimers Dis Other Demen, 29*, 76-83.

[26] Wu, J., Basha, M. R., Brock, B., Cox, D. P., Cardozo-Pelaez, F., McPherson, C. A., Harry, J., et al. (2008). Alzheimer's disease (AD)-like pathology in aged monkeys after infantile exposure to environmental metal lead (Pb): evidence for a developmental origin and environmental link for AD. *J Neurosci, 28*, 3-9.

[27] Bihaqi, S. W. & Zawia, N. H. (2012). Alzheimer's disease biomarkers and epigenetic intermediates following exposure to Pb in vitro. *Curr Alzheimer Res, 9*, 555-562.

[28] Huang, H., Bihaqi, S. W., Cui, L. & Zawia, N. H. (2011). In vitro Pb exposure disturbs the balance between Abeta production and elimination: the role of AbetaPP and neprilysin. *Neurotoxicology, 32*, 300-306.

[29] Coon, S., Stark, A., Peterson, E., Gloi, A., Kortsha, G., Pounds, J., Chettle, D., et al. (2006). Whole-body lifetime occupational lead exposure and risk of Parkinson's disease. *Environ Health Perspect, 114,* 1872-1876.

[30] Kala, S. V. & Jadhav, A. L. (1995). Low level lead exposure decreases in vivo release of dopamine in the rat nucleus accumbens: a microdialysis study. *J Neurochem, 65,* 1631-1635.

[31] Yamin, G., Glaser, C. B., Uversky, V. N. & Fink, A. L. (2003). Certain metals trigger fibrillation of methionine-oxidized alpha-synuclein. *J Biol Chem, 278,* 27630-27635.

[32] Kamel, F., Umbach, D. M., Hu, H., Munsat, T. L., Shefner, J. M., Taylor, J. A. & Sandler, D. P. (2005). Lead exposure as a risk factor for amyotrophic lateral sclerosis. *Neurodegener Dis, 2,* 195-201.

[33] Wang, M. D., Gomes, J., Cashman, N. R., Little, J. & Krewski, D. (2014). A meta-analysis of observational studies of the association between chronic occupational exposure to lead and amyotrophic lateral sclerosis. *J Occup Environ Med, 56,* 1235-1242.

[34] Marques, S. C., Oliveira, C. R., Pereira, C. M. & Outeiro, T. F. (2011). Epigenetics in neurodegeneration: a new layer of complexity. *Prog Neuropsychopharmacol Biol Psychiatry, 35,* 348-355.

[35] Block, M. L. & Hong, J. S. (2005). Microglia and inflammation-mediated neurodegeneration: multiple triggers with a common mechanism. *Prog Neurobiol, 76,* 77-98.

[36] Dickens, A. M., Vainio, S., Marjamaki, P., Johansson, J., Lehtiniemi, P., Rokka, J., Rinne, J., et al. (2014). Detection of microglial activation in an acute model of neuroinflammation using PET and radiotracers 11C-(R)-PK11195 and 18F-GE-180. *J Nucl Med, 55,* 466-472.

[37] Schindler, S. M., Spielman, L. J., E., B., Slattery, W. T., Harris, D. B. & Klegeris, A., *The Diversity of Microglial Activators and Their Elicited Responses: Implications for Central Nervous System Functions,* in *Microglia: Physiology, Regulation and Health Implications,* E.R. Giffard, Editor 2015, Nova Science Publishers: Hauppauge, NY.

[38] Dheen, S. T., Kaur, C. & Ling, E. A. (2007). Microglial activation and its implications in the brain diseases. *Curr Med Chem, 14,* 1189-1197.

[39] Lull, M. E. & Block, M. L. (2010). Microglial activation and chronic neurodegeneration. *Neurotherapeutics, 7,* 354-65.

[40] Frank-Cannon, T. C., Alto, L. T., McAlpine, F. E. & Tansey, M. G. (2009). Does neuroinflammation fan the flame in neurodegenerative diseases? *Mol Neurodegener, 4,* 1-13.

[41] Block, M. L., Zecca, L. & Hong, J. S. (2007). Microglia-mediated neurotoxicity: uncovering the molecular mechanisms. *Nat Rev Neurosci*, *8*, 57-69.

[42] Colton, C. A. (2009). Heterogeneity of Microglial Activation in the Innate Immune Response in the Brain. *J Neuroimmune Pharmacol*, *4*, 399-418.

[43] Minghetti, L., Ajmone-Cat, M. A., De Berardinis, M. A. & De Simone, R. (2005). Microglial activation in chronic neurodegenerative diseases: roles of apoptotic neurons and chronic stimulation. *Brain Res Brain Res Rev*, *48*, 251-256.

[44] McGeer, P. L. & McGeer, E. G. (2002). Inflammatory processes in amyotrophic lateral sclerosis. *Muscle Nerve*, *26*, 459-470.

[45] Wyss-Coray, T. (2006). Inflammation in Alzheimer disease: driving force, bystander or beneficial response? *Nat Med*, *12*, 1005-1015.

[46] Akiyama, H., Mori, H., Saido, T., Kondo, H., Ikeda, K. & McGeer, P. L. (1999). Occurrence of the diffuse amyloid beta-protein (Abeta) deposits with numerous Abeta-containing glial cells in the cerebral cortex of patients with Alzheimer's disease. *Glia*, *25*, 324-331.

[47] Barcia, C., Ros, F., Carrillo, M. A., Aguado-Llera, D., Ros, C. M., Gomez, A., Nombela, C., et al. (2009). Inflammatory response in Parkinsonism. *J Neural Transm Suppl*, *73*, 245-252.

[48] Rosen, D. R., Siddique, T., Patterson, D., Figlewicz, D. A., Sapp, P., Hentati, A., Donaldson, D., et al. (1993). Mutations in Cu/Zn superoxide dismutase gene are associated with familial amyotrophic lateral sclerosis. *Nature*, *362*, 59-62.

[49] Glass, C. K., Saijo, K., Winner, B., Marchetto, M. C. & Gage, F. H. (2010). Mechanisms underlying inflammation in neurodegeneration. *Cell*, *140*, 918-934.

[50] Gibbons, H. M. & Dragunow, M. (2006). Microglia induce neural cell death via a proximity-dependent mechanism involving nitric oxide. *Brain Res*, *1084*, 1-15.

[51] Combs, C. K., Karlo, J. C., Kao, S. C. & Landreth, G. E. (2001). beta-Amyloid stimulation of microglia and monocytes results in TNFalpha-dependent expression of inducible nitric oxide synthase and neuronal apoptosis. *J Neurosci 21*, 1179-1188.

[52] Dheen, S. T., Jun, Y., Yan, Z., Tay, S. S. & Ling, E. A. (2005). Retinoic acid inhibits expression of TNF-alpha and iNOS in activated rat microglia. *Glia*, *50*, 21-31.

[53] Qin, L., Liu, Y., Cooper, C., Liu, B., Wilson, B. & Hong, J. S. (2002). Microglia enhance beta-amyloid peptide-induced toxicity in cortical and mesencephalic neurons by producing reactive oxygen species. *J Neurochem, 83,* 973-983.

[54] Smits, H. A., Rijsmus, A., van Loon, J. H., Wat, J. W., Verhoef, J., Boven, L. A. & Nottet, H. S. (2002). Amyloid-beta-induced chemokine production in primary human macrophages and astrocytes. *J Neuroimmunol, 127,* 160-168.

[55] Walker, D. G., Link, J., Lue, L. F., Dalsing-Hernandez, J. E. & Boyes, B. E. (2006). Gene expression changes by amyloid beta peptide-stimulated human postmortem brain microglia identify activation of multiple inflammatory processes. *J Leukoc Biol, 79,* 596-610.

[56] Walker, D. G., Lue, L. F. & Beach, T. G. (2001). Gene expression profiling of amyloid beta peptide-stimulated human post-mortem brain microglia. *Neurobiol Aging, 22,* 957-966.

[57] McGeer, P. L., Itagaki, S., Boyes, B. E. & McGeer, E. G. (1988). Reactive microglia are positive for HLA-DR in the substantia nigra of Parkinson's and Alzheimer's disease brains. *Neurology, 38,* 1285-1291.

[58] Gerhard, A., Pavese, N., Hotton, G., Turkheimer, F., Es, M., Hammers, A., Eggert, K., et al. (2006). In vivo imaging of microglial activation with [11C](R)-PK11195 PET in idiopathic Parkinson's disease. *Neurobiol Dis, 21,* 404-412.

[59] Gerhard, A. (2013). Imaging of neuroinflammation in parkinsonian syndromes with positron emission tomography. *Curr Neurol Neurosci Rep, 13,* 405.

[60] Hunot, S., Dugas, N., Faucheux, B., Hartmann, A., Tardieu, M., Debre, P., Agid, Y., et al. (1999). FcepsilonRII/CD23 is expressed in Parkinson's disease and induces, in vitro, production of nitric oxide and tumor necrosis factor-alpha in glial cells. *J Neurosci, 19,* 3440-3447.

[61] Nagatsu, T. & Sawada, M. (2005). Inflammatory process in Parkinson's disease: role for cytokines. *Curr Pharm Des, 11,* 999-1016.

[62] Zhang, W., Wang, T., Pei, Z., Miller, D. S., Wu, X., Block, M. L., Wilson, B., et al. (2005). Aggregated alpha-synuclein activates microglia: a process leading to disease progression in Parkinson's disease. *FASEB J, 19,* 533-542.

[63] Harms, A. S., Cao, S., Rowse, A. L., Thome, A. D., Li, X., Mangieri, L. R., Cron, R. Q., et al. (2013). MHCII is required for alpha-synuclein-induced activation of microglia, CD4 T cell proliferation, and dopaminergic neurodegeneration. *J Neurosci, 33,* 9592-9600.

[64] Sacino, A. N., Brooks, M., McKinney, A. B., Thomas, M. A., Shaw, G., Golde, T. E. & Giasson, B. I. (2014). Brain Injection of alpha-Synuclein Induces Multiple Proteinopathies, Gliosis, and a Neuronal Injury Marker. *J Neurosci, 34,* 12368-12378.

[65] Schapansky, J., Nardozzi, J. D. & LaVoie, M. J. (2014). The complex relationships between microglia, alpha-synuclein, and LRRK2 in Parkinson's disease. *Neuroscience, 14,* 1-15.

[66] Klegeris, A., Pelech, S., Giasson, B. I., Maguire, J., Zhang, H., McGeer, E. G. & McGeer, P. L. (2008). alpha-Synuclein activates stress signaling protein kinases in THP-1 cells and microglia. *Neurobiol Aging 29,* 739-752.

[67] Zhang, W., Dallas, S., Zhang, D., Guo, J. P., Pang, H., Wilson, B., Miller, D. S., et al. (2007). Microglial PHOX and Mac-1 are essential to the enhanced dopaminergic neurodegeneration elicited by A30P and A53T mutant alpha-synuclein. *Glia, 55,* 1178-1188.

[68] Turner, M. R., Cagnin, A., Turkheimer, F. E., Miller, C. C., Shaw, C. E., Brooks, D. J., Leigh, P. N., et al. (2004). Evidence of widespread cerebral microglial activation in amyotrophic lateral sclerosis: an [11C](R)-PK11195 positron emission tomography study. *Neurobiol Dis, 15,* 601-609.

[69] Zurcher, N. R., Loggia, M. L., Lawson, R., Chonde, D. B., Izquierdo-Garcia, D., Yasek, J. E., Akeju, O., et al. (2015). Increased in vivo glial activation in patients with amyotrophic lateral sclerosis: assessed with [(11)C]-PBR28. *Neuroimage Clin, 7,* 409-414.

[70] Kuhle, J., Lindberg, R. L., Regeniter, A., Mehling, M., Steck, A. J., Kappos, L. & Czaplinski, A. (2009). Increased levels of inflammatory chemokines in amyotrophic lateral sclerosis. *Eur J Neurol, 16,* 771-774.

[71] Henkel, J. S., Engelhardt, J. I., Siklos, L., Simpson, E. P., Kim, S. H., Pan, T., Goodman, J. C., et al. (2004). Presence of dendritic cells, MCP-1, and activated microglia/macrophages in amyotrophic lateral sclerosis spinal cord tissue. *Ann Neurol, 55,* 221-235.

[72] Galland, L. (2010). Diet and Inflammation. *Nutr Clin Pract, 25,* 634-640.

[73] Russo, G. L. (2009). Dietary n − 6 and n − 3 polyunsaturated fatty acids: From biochemistry to clinical implications in cardiovascular prevention. *Biochem Pharmacol, 77,* 937-946.

[74] Simopoulos, A. P. (2006). Evolutionary aspects of diet, the omega-6/omega-3 ratio and genetic variation: nutritional implications for chronic diseases. *Biomed Pharmacother, 60,* 502-507.

[75] Franzen-Castle, L. D. (2010). Omega-3 and Omega-6 Fatty Acids. *NIANR*, 1-4.

[76] Cunnane, S. C. (2003). Problems with essential fatty acids: time for a new paradigm? *Prog Lipid Res*, *42*, 544-568.

[77] Sijben, J. W. C. & Calder, P. C. (2007). Differential immunomodulation with long-chain n-3 PUFA in health and chronic disease. *Proc Nutr Soc*, *66*, 237-259.

[78] Peterson, L. D., Jeffery, N. M., Thies, F., Sanderson, P., Newsholme, E. A. & Calder, P. C. (1998). Eicosapentaenoic and docosahexaenoic acids alter rat spleen leukocyte fatty acid composition and prostaglandin E2 production but have different effects on lymphocyte functions and cell-mediated immunity. *Lipids*, *33*, 171-180.

[79] Legler, D. F., Bruckner, M., Uetz-von Allmen, E. & Krause, P. (2010). Prostaglandin E2 at new glance: novel insights in functional diversity offer therapeutic chances. *Int J Biochem Cell Biol*, *42*, 198-201.

[80] Cole, G. M., Ma, Q. L. & Frautschy, S. A. (2010). Dietary fatty acids and the aging brain. *Nutr Rev*, *68*, S102-S111.

[81] Burdge, G. C. & Calder, P. C. (2005). Conversion of α-linolenic acid to longer-chain polyunsaturated fatty acids in human adults. *Reprod Nutr Dev*, *45*, 581-597.

[82] Calder, P. C. (2006). Polyunsaturated fatty acids and inflammation. *Prostaglandins Leukot Essent Fatty Acids*, *75*, 197-202.

[83] Calder, P. C. (2006). n-3 polyunsaturated fatty acids, inflammation, and inflammatory diseases. *Am J Clin Nutr*, *83*, 1505S-1519S.

[84] Matsusaka, T., Fujikawa, K., Nishio, Y., Mukaida, N., Matsushima, K., Kishimoto, T. & Akira, S. (1993). Transcription factors NF-IL6 and NF-kappa B synergistically activate transcription of the inflammatory cytokines, interleukin 6 and interleukin 8. *Proc Natl Acad Sci USA 90*, 10193-10197.

[85] Hayden, M. S. & Ghosh, S. (2011). NF-κB in immunobiology. *Cell Res 21*, 223-244.

[86] Pischon, T., Hankinson, S. E., Hotamisligil, G. S., Rifai, N., Willett, W. C. & Rimm, E. B. (2003). Habitual dietary intake of n-3 and n-6 fatty acids in relation to inflammatory markers among US men and women. *Circulation*, *108*, 155-160.

[87] Ikemoto, A., Ohishi, M., Sato, Y., Hata, N., Misawa, Y., Fujii, Y. & Okuyama, H. (2001). Reversibility of n-3 fatty acid deficiency-induced alterations of learning behavior in the rat: level of n-6 fatty acids as another critical factor. *J Lipid Res*, *42*, 1655-1663.

[88] Morris, M. C. (2003). Consumption of fish and n-3 fatty acids and risk of incident Alzheimer disease. *JAMA*, *290*, 2104.

[89] Orr, S. K., Trepanier, M. O. & Bazinet, R. P. (2013). n-3 Polyunsaturated fatty acids in animal models with neuroinflammation. *Prostaglandins Leukot Essent Fatty Acids*, *88*, 97-103.

[90] Zendedel, A., Habib, P., Dang, J., Lammerding, L., Hoffmann, S., Beyer, C. & Slowik, A. (2015). Omega-3 polyunsaturated fatty acids ameliorate neuroinflammation and mitigate ischemic stroke damage through interactions with astrocytes and microglia. *J Neuroimmunol*, *278*, 200-211.

[91] Uttara, B., Singh, A., Zamboni, P. & Mahajan, R. (2009). Oxidative Stress and Neurodegenerative Diseases: A Review of Upstream and Downstream Antioxidant Therapeutic Options. *Curr Neuropharmacol*, *7*, 65-74.

[92] Pandey, K. B. & Rizvi, S. I. (2009). Plant polyphenols as dietary antioxidants in human health and disease. *Oxid Med Cell Longev*, *2*, 270-278.

[93] Lau, F. C., Bielinski, D. F. & Joseph, J. A. (2007). Inhibitory effects of blueberry extract on the production of inflammatory mediators in lipopolysaccharide activated BV2 microglia. *J Neurosci Res*, *85*, 1010-1017.

[94] Poulose, S. M., Fisher, D. R., Larson, J., Bielinski, D. F., Rimando, A. M., Carey, A. N., Schauss, A. G., et al. (2012). Anthocyanin-rich açai (Euterpe oleracea Mart.) fruit pulp fractions attenuate inflammatory stress signaling in mouse brain BV-2 microglial cells. *J Agric Food Chem*, *60*, 1084.

[95] Frautschy, S. A., Hu, W., Kim, P., Miller, S. A., Chu, T., Harris-White, M. E. & Cole, G. M. (2001). Phenolic anti-inflammatory antioxidant reversal of Abeta-induced cognitive deficits and neuropathology. *Neurobiol Aging*, *22*, 993.

[96] Ganguli, M., Chandra, V., Kamboh, I. & Johnston, J. M. (2000). Apoplipoprotein E Polymorphism and Alzheimer disease: The indo-US cross-national dementia study. *Arch Neurol*, *57*, 824.

[97] Schardt, D. (2012). Caffeine. *Nutrition Action Health Letter*, *39*, 7.

[98] Bailey, R. L., Saldanha, L. G., Gahche, J. J. & Dwyer, J. T. (2014). Estimating caffeine intake from energy drinks and dietary supplements in the United States. *Nutr Rev*, *72*, 9-13.

[99] Kalda, A., Yu, L., Oztas, E. & Chen, J. F. (2006). Novel neuroprotection by caffeine and adenosine A(2A) receptor antagonists in animal models of Parkinson's disease. *J Neurol Sci, 248*, 9.

[100] Nobre, J. H. V., Cunha, G. M. d. A., de Vasconcelos, L. M., Magalhães, H. I. F., Oliveira Neto, R. N., Maia, F. D., de Moraes, M. O., et al. (2010). Caffeine and CSC, adenosine A2A antagonists, offer neuroprotection against 6-OHDA-induced neurotoxicity in rat mesencephalic cells. *Neurochem Int, 56*, 51-58.

[101] Sonsalla, P. K., Wong, L.-Y., Harris, S. L., Richardson, J. R., Khobahy, I., Li, W., Gadad, B. S., et al. (2012). Delayed caffeine treatment prevents nigral dopamine neuron loss in a progressive rat model of Parkinson's disease. *Exp Neurol, 234*, 482-487.

[102] Kang, C.-H., Jayasooriya, R. G. P. T., Dilshara, M. G., Choi, Y. H., Jeong, Y.-K., Kim, N. D. & Kim, G.-Y. (2012). Caffeine suppresses lipopolysaccharide-stimulated BV2 microglial cells by suppressing Akt-mediated NF-κB activation and ERK phosphorylation. *Food Chem Toxicol, 50*, 4270-4276.

[103] Fiebich, B. L., Lieb, K., Hüll, M., Aicher, B., van Ryn, J., Pairet, M. & Engelhardt, G. (2000). Effects of caffeine and paracetamol alone or in combination with acetylsalicylic acid on prostaglandin E2 synthesis in rat microglial cells. *Neuropharmacology, 39*, 2205-2213.

[104] Chen, X., Lan, X., Roche, I., Liu, R. & Geiger, J. D. (2008). Caffeine protects against MPTP induced blood brain barrier dysfunction in mouse striatum. *J Neurochem, 107*, 1147-1157.

[105] Ujiie, M., Dickstein, D. L., Carlow, D. A. & Jefferies, W. A. (2003). Blood—Brain Barrier Permeability Precedes Senile Plaque Formation in an Alzheimer Disease Model. *Microcirculation, 10*, 463-470.

[106] Stewart, L. K., Flynn, M. G., Campbell, W. W., Craig, B. A., Robinson, J. P., McFarlin, B. K., Timmerman, K. L., et al. (2005). Influence of exercise training and age on CD14+ cell-surface expression of toll-like receptor 2 and 4. *Brain Behav Immun, 19*, 389-397.

[107] Peixoto, T. C., Begot, I., Bolzan, D. W., Machado, L., Reis, M. S., Papa, V., Carvalho, A. C., et al. (2015). Early exercise-based rehabilitation improves health-related quality of life and functional capacity after acute myocardial infarction: a randomized controlled trial. *Can J Cardiol, 31*, 308-313.

[108] Moore, S. A., Hallsworth, K., Jakovljevic, D. G., Blamire, A. M., He, J., Ford, G. A., Rochester, L., et al. (2014). Effects of Community Exercise Therapy on Metabolic, Brain, Physical, and Cognitive Function

Following Stroke: A Randomized Controlled Pilot Trial. *Neurorehabil Neural Repair*, *1545968314562116*,

[109] Stojanovic, M. D., Ostojic, S. M., Calleja-Gonzalez, J., Milosevic, Z. & Mikic, M. (2012). Correlation between explosive strength, aerobic power and repeated sprint ability in elite basketball players. *J Sports Med Phys Fitness*, *52*, 375-381.

[110] Egan, B. & Zierath, J. R. (2013). Exercise metabolism and the molecular regulation of skeletal muscle adaptation. *Cell Metab*, *17*, 162-184.

[111] Gleeson, M., Bishop, N. C., Stensel, D. J., Lindley, M. R., Mastana, S. S. & Nimmo, M. A. (2011). The anti-inflammatory effects of exercise: mechanisms and implications for the prevention and treatment of disease. *Nat Rev Immunol*, *11*, 607-615.

[112] Flynn, M. G. & McFarlin, B. K. (2006). Toll-like receptor 4: link to the anti-inflammatory effects of exercise? *Exerc Sport Sci Rev*, *34*, 176-181.

[113] Pedersen, B. K. (2006). The anti-inflammatory effect of exercise: its role in diabetes and cardiovascular disease control. *Essays Biochem*, *42*, 105-117.

[114] Starkie, R., Ostrowski, S. R., Jauffred, S., Febbraio, M. & Pedersen, B. K. (2003). Exercise and IL-6 infusion inhibit endotoxin-induced TNF-alpha production in humans. *FASEB J*, *17*, 884-886.

[115] McFarlin, B. K., Flynn, M. G., Campbell, W. W., Craig, B. A., Robinson, J. P., Stewart, L. K., Timmerman, K. L., et al. (2006). Physical activity status, but not age, influences inflammatory biomarkers and toll-like receptor 4. *J Gerontol A Biol Sci Med Sci*, *61*, 388-393.

[116] Steensberg, A., Fischer, C. P., Keller, C., Moller, K. & Pedersen, B. K. (2003). IL-6 enhances plasma IL-1ra, IL-10, and cortisol in humans. *Am J Physiol Endocrinol Metab*, *285*, E433-437.

[117] Oliveira, A. G., Araujo, T. G., Carvalho, B. M., Guadagnini, D., Rocha, G. Z., Bagarolli, R. A., Carvalheira, J. B., et al. (2013). Acute exercise induces a phenotypic switch in adipose tissue macrophage polarization in diet-induced obese rats. *Obesity 21*, 2545-2556.

[118] Bruun, J. M., Helge, J. W., Richelsen, B. & Stallknecht, B. (2006). Diet and exercise reduce low-grade inflammation and macrophage infiltration in adipose tissue but not in skeletal muscle in severely obese subjects. *Am J Physiol Endocrinol Metab*, *290*, E961-967.

[119] Gleeson, M., McFarlin, B. & Flynn, M. (2006). Exercise and Toll-like receptors. *Exerc Immunol Rev*, *12*, 34-53.

[120] Oliveira, A. G., Carvalho, B. M., Tobar, N., Ropelle, E. R., Pauli, J. R., Bagarolli, R. A., Guadagnini, D., et al. (2011). Physical exercise reduces

circulating lipopolysaccharide and TLR4 activation and improves insulin signaling in tissues of DIO rats. *Diabetes*, *60*, 784-796.

[121] Kohman, R. A., DeYoung, E. K., Bhattacharya, T. K., Peterson, L. N. & Rhodes, J. S. (2012). Wheel running attenuates microglia proliferation and increases expression of a proneurogenic phenotype in the hippocampus of aged mice. *Brain Behav Immun*, *26*, 803-810.

[122] Funk, J. A., Gohlke, J., Kraft, A. D., McPherson, C. A., Collins, J. B. & Jean Harry, G. (2011). Voluntary exercise protects hippocampal neurons from trimethyltin injury: possible role of interleukin-6 to modulate tumor necrosis factor receptor-mediated neurotoxicity. *Brain Behav Immun*, *25*, 1063-1077.

[123] Leem, Y. H., Lee, Y. I., Son, H. J. & Lee, S. H. (2011). Chronic exercise ameliorates the neuroinflammation in mice carrying NSE/htau23. *Biochem Biophys Res Commun*, *406*, 359-365.

[124] Nichol, K. E., Poon, W. W., Parachikova, A. I., Cribbs, D. H., Glabe, C. G. & Cotman, C. W. (2008). Exercise alters the immune profile in Tg2576 Alzheimer mice toward a response coincident with improved cognitive performance and decreased amyloid. *J Neuroinflammation*, *5*, 13.

[125] Piao, C. S., Stoica, B. A., Wu, J., Sabirzhanov, B., Zhao, Z., Cabatbat, R., Loane, D. J., et al. (2013). Late exercise reduces neuroinflammation and cognitive dysfunction after traumatic brain injury. *Neurobiol Dis*, *54*, 252-263.

[126] Barnes, D. E. & Yaffe, K. (2011). The projected effect of risk factor reduction on Alzheimer's disease prevalence. *Lancet Neurol*, *10*, 819-828.

[127] Zou, Y. M., Tan, J. P., Li, N., Yang, J. S., Yu, B. C., Yu, J. M., Zhao, Y. M., et al. (2015). Do physical exercise and reading reduce the risk of Parkinson's disease? a cross-sectional study on factors associated with Parkinson's disease in elderly Chinese veterans. *Neuropsychiatr Dis Treat*, *11*, 695-700.

[128] Bello-Haas, V. D., Florence, J. M., Kloos, A. D., Scheirbecker, J., Lopate, G., Hayes, S. M., Pioro, E. P., et al. (2007). A randomized controlled trial of resistance exercise in individuals with ALS. *Neurology*, *68*, 2003-2007.

[129] Allison, D. J. & Ditor, D. S. (2014). The common inflammatory etiology of depression and cognitive impairment: a therapeutic target. *J Neuroinflammation*, *11*, 1-12.

[130] Spielman, L. J., Little, J. P. & Klegeris, A. (2014). Inflammation and insulin/IGF-1 resistance as the possible link between obesity and neurodegeneration. *J Neuroimmunol, 273*, 8-21.

[131] Meeusen, R. (2014). Exercise, nutrition and the brain. *Sports Med, 44 Suppl 1*, S47-56.

[132] Gavett, B. E., Stern, R. A., Cantu, R. C., Nowinski, C. J. & McKee, A. C. (2010). Mild traumatic brain injury: a risk factor for neurodegeneration. *Alzheimers Res Ther, 2*, 18.

[133] Mortimer, J. A., van Duijn, C. M., Chandra, V., Fratiglioni, L., Graves, A. B., Heyman, A., Jorm, A. F., et al. (1991). Head trauma as a risk factor for Alzheimer's disease: a collaborative re-analysis of case-control studies. EURODEM Risk Factors Research Group. *Int J Epidemiol, 20 Suppl 2*, S28-35.

[134] Goldman, S. M., Tanner, C. M., Oakes, D., Bhudhikanok, G. S., Gupta, A. & Langston, J. W. (2006). Head injury and Parkinson's disease risk in twins. *Ann Neurol, 60*, 65-72.

[135] Chen, H., Richard, M., Sandler, D. P., Umbach, D. M. & Kamel, F. (2007). Head injury and amyotrophic lateral sclerosis. *Am J Epidemiol, 166*, 810-816.

[136] Lozano, D., Gonzales-Portillo, G. S., Acosta, S., de la Pena, I., Tajiri, N., Kaneko, Y. & Borlongan, C. V. (2015). Neuroinflammatory responses to traumatic brain injury: etiology, clinical consequences, and therapeutic opportunities. *Neuropsychiatr Dis Treat, 11*, 97-106.

[137] Faden, A. I. & Loane, D. J. (2015). Chronic neurodegeneration after traumatic brain injury: Alzheimer disease, chronic traumatic encephalopathy, or persistent neuroinflammation? *Neurotherapeutics, 12*, 143-150.

[138] Breunig, J. J., Guillot-Sestier, M. V. & Town, T. (2013). Brain injury, neuroinflammation and Alzheimer's disease. *Front Aging Neurosci, 5*, 26.

[139] Kumar, A. & Loane, D. J. (2012). Neuroinflammation after traumatic brain injury: opportunities for therapeutic intervention. *Brain Behav Immun, 26*, 1191-201.

[140] McIntosh, T. K., Smith, D. H., Meaney, D. F., Kotapka, M. J., Gennarelli, T. A. & Graham, D. I. (1996). Neuropathological sequelae of traumatic brain injury: relationship to neurochemical and biomechanical mechanisms. *Lab Invest, 74*, 315-342.

[141] Yakovlev, A. G., Knoblach, S. M., Fan, L., Fox, G. B., Goodnight, R. & Faden, A. I. (1997). Activation of CPP32-like caspases contributes to

neuronal apoptosis and neurological dysfunction after traumatic brain injury. *J Neurosci, 17*, 7415-7424.

[142] Gentile, N. T. & McIntosh, T. K. (1993). Antagonists of excitatory amino acids and endogenous opioid peptides in the treatment of experimental central nervous system injury. *Ann Emerg Med, 22*, 1028-34.

[143] Faden, A. I., Demediuk, P., Panter, S. S. & Vink, R. (1989). The role of excitatory amino acids and NMDA receptors in traumatic brain injury. *Science, 244*, 798-800.

[144] Xiong, Y., Gu, Q., Peterson, P. L., Muizelaar, J. P. & Lee, C. P. (1997). Mitochondrial dysfunction and calcium perturbation induced by traumatic brain injury. *J Neurotrauma, 14*, 23-34.

[145] Morganti-Kossmann, M. C., Satgunaseelan, L., Bye, N. & Kossmann, T. (2007). Modulation of immune response by head injury. *Injury, 38*, 1392-1400.

[146] Sundman, M. H., Hall, E. E. & Chen, N. K. (2014). Examining the relationship between head trauma and neurodegenerative disease: A review of epidemiology, pathology and neuroimaging techniques. *J Alzheimers Dis Parkinsonism, 4*, 1-47.

[147] Ziebell, J. M. & Morganti-Kossmann, M. C. (2010). Involvement of pro- and anti-inflammatory cytokines and chemokines in the pathophysiology of traumatic brain injury. *Neurotherapeutics, 7*, 22-30.

[148] Loane, D. J. & Byrnes, K. R. (2010). Role of microglia in neurotrauma. *Neurotherapeutics, 7*, 366-377.

[149] Simard, J. M., Kahle, K. T. & Gerzanich, V. (2010). Molecular mechanisms of microvascular failure in central nervous system injury--synergistic roles of NKCC1 and SUR1/TRPM4. *J Neurosurg, 113*, 622-629.

[150] Johnson, V. E., Stewart, J. E., Begbie, F. D., Trojanowski, J. Q., Smith, D. H. & Stewart, W. (2013). Inflammation and white matter degeneration persist for years after a single traumatic brain injury. *Brain, 136*, 28-42.

[151] Gentleman, S. M., Leclercq, P. D., Moyes, L., Graham, D. I., Smith, C., Griffin, W. S. & Nicoll, J. A. (2004). Long-term intracerebral inflammatory response after traumatic brain injury. *Forensic Sci Int, 146*, 97-104.

[152] Israelsson, C., Bengtsson, H., Kylberg, A., Kullander, K., Lewen, A., Hillered, L. & Ebendal, T. (2008). Distinct cellular patterns of

upregulated chemokine expression supporting a prominent inflammatory role in traumatic brain injury. *J Neurotrauma, 25*, 959-974.

[153] Davalos, D., Grutzendler, J., Yang, G., Kim, J. V., Zuo, Y., Jung, S., Littman, D. R., et al. (2005). ATP mediates rapid microglial response to local brain injury in vivo. *Nat Neurosci, 8*, 752-758.

[154] Csuka, E., Morganti-Kossmann, M. C., Lenzlinger, P. M., Joller, H., Trentz, O. & Kossmann, T. (1999). IL-10 levels in cerebrospinal fluid and serum of patients with severe traumatic brain injury: relationship to IL-6, TNF-alpha, TGF-beta1 and blood-brain barrier function. *J Neuroimmunol, 101*, 211-221.

[155] Morganti-Kossmann, M. C., Hans, V. H., Lenzlinger, P. M., Dubs, R., Ludwig, E., Trentz, O. & Kossmann, T. (1999). TGF-beta is elevated in the CSF of patients with severe traumatic brain injuries and parallels blood-brain barrier function. *J Neurotrauma, 16*, 617-628.

[156] Holmin, S. & Mathiesen, T. (1999). Long-term intracerebral inflammatory response after experimental focal brain injury in rat. *Neuroreport, 10*, 1889-1891.

[157] Smith, D. H., Chen, X. H., Pierce, J. E., Wolf, J. A., Trojanowski, J. Q., Graham, D. I. & McIntosh, T. K. (1997). Progressive atrophy and neuron death for one year following brain trauma in the rat. *J Neurotrauma, 14*, 715-727.

[158] Tang, D., Kang, R., Coyne, C. B., Zeh, H. J. & Lotze, M. T. (2012). PAMPs and DAMPs: signal 0s that spur autophagy and immunity. *Immunol Rev, 249*, 158-75.

[159] Srikrishna, G. & Freeze, H. H. (2009). Endogenous damage-associated molecular pattern molecules at the crossroads of inflammation and cancer. *Neoplasia, 11*, 615-628.

[160] Wu, L. J., Vadakkan, K. I. & Zhuo, M. (2007). ATP-induced chemotaxis of microglial processes requires P2Y receptor-activated initiation of outward potassium currents. *Glia, 55*, 810-821.

[161] Taylor, D. L., Jones, F., Kubota, E. S. & Pocock, J. M. (2005). Stimulation of microglial metabotropic glutamate receptor mGlu2 triggers tumor necrosis factor alpha-induced neurotoxicity in concert with microglial-derived Fas ligand. *J Neurosci, 25*, 2952-2964.

[162] Solito, E. & Sastre, M. (2012). Microglia function in Alzheimer's disease. *Front Pharmacol, 3*, 14.

[163] Bramlett, H. M. & Dietrich, W. D. (2002). Quantitative structural changes in white and gray matter 1 year following traumatic brain injury in rats. *Acta Neuropathol, 103*, 607-614.

[164] Chao, C. C., Hu, S., Ehrlich, L. & Peterson, P. K. (1995). Interleukin-1 and tumor necrosis factor-alpha synergistically mediate neurotoxicity: involvement of nitric oxide and of N-methyl-D-aspartate receptors. *Brain Behav Immun, 9*, 355-365.

[165] Goodman, J. C., Robertson, C. S., Grossman, R. G. & Narayan, R. K. (1990). Elevation of tumor necrosis factor in head injury. *J Neuroimmunol, 30*, 213-217.

[166] Woodroofe, M. N., Sarna, G. S., Wadhwa, M., Hayes, G. M., Loughlin, A. J., Tinker, A. & Cuzner, M. L. (1991). Detection of interleukin-1 and interleukin-6 in adult rat brain, following mechanical injury, by in vivo microdialysis: evidence of a role for microglia in cytokine production. *J Neuroimmunol, 33*, 227-236.

[167] Winter, C. D., Iannotti, F., Pringle, A. K., Trikkas, C., Clough, G. F. & Church, M. K. (2002). A microdialysis method for the recovery of IL-1beta, IL-6 and nerve growth factor from human brain in vivo. *J Neurosci Methods, 119*, 45-50.

[168] Stover, J. F., Schoning, B., Beyer, T. F., Woiciechowsky, C. & Unterberg, A. W. (2000). Temporal profile of cerebrospinal fluid glutamate, interleukin-6, and tumor necrosis factor-alpha in relation to brain edema and contusion following controlled cortical impact injury in rats. *Neurosci Lett, 288*, 25-28.

[169] Morganti-Kossmann, M. C., Rancan, M., Otto, V. I., Stahel, P. F. & Kossmann, T. (2001). Role of cerebral inflammation after traumatic brain injury: a revisited concept. *Shock, 16*, 165-177.

[170] Saw, M. M., Chamberlain, J., Barr, M., Morgan, M. P., Burnett, J. R. & Ho, K. M. (2014). Differential disruption of blood-brain barrier in severe traumatic brain injury. *Neurocrit Care, 20*, 209-216.

[171] Utagawa, A., Truettner, J. S., Dietrich, W. D. & Bramlett, H. M. (2008). Systemic inflammation exacerbates behavioral and histopathological consequences of isolated traumatic brain injury in rats. *Exp Neurol, 211*, 283-291.

[172] Das, M., Mohapatra, S. & Mohapatra, S. S. (2012). New perspectives on central and peripheral immune responses to acute traumatic brain injury. *J Neuroinflammation, 9*, 236.

[173] Mouzon, B. C., Bachmeier, C., Ferro, A., Ojo, J. O., Crynen, G., Acker, C. M., Davies, P., et al. (2014). Chronic neuropathological and neurobehavioral changes in a repetitive mild traumatic brain injury model. *Ann Neurol, 75*, 241-254.

[174] Aungst, S. L., Kabadi, S. V., Thompson, S. M., Stoica, B. A. & Faden, A. I. (2014). Repeated mild traumatic brain injury causes chronic neuroinflammation, changes in hippocampal synaptic plasticity, and associated cognitive deficits. *J Cereb Blood Flow Metab, 34*, 1223-1232.

[175] Gustafson, D., Rothenberg, E., Blennow, K., Steen, B. & Skoog, I. (2003). An 18-year follow-up of overweight and risk of Alzheimer disease. *Arch Intern Med, 163*, 1524-1528.

[176] Viticchi, G., Falsetti, L., Buratti, L., Luzzi, S., Bartolini, M., Acciarri, M. C., Provinciali, L., et al. (2015). Metabolic syndrome and cerebrovascular impairment in Alzheimer's disease. *Int J Geriatr Psychiatry, 4269*, 1-6.

[177] Kaur, J. (2014). A comprehensive review on metabolic syndrome. *Cardiol Res Pract, 2014*, 943162.

[178] World Health Organization (2014). Obesity and overweight. *Fact Sheet No 311*, [cited July 30, 2014].

[179] Costanzo, P., Cleland, J. G., Pellicori, P., Clark, A. L., Hepburn, D., Kilpatrick, E. S., Perrone-Filardi, P., et al. (2015). The obesity paradox in type 2 diabetes mellitus: relationship of body mass index to prognosis: a cohort study. *Ann Intern Med, 162*, 610-618.

[180] Gustafson, D. R., Backman, K., Joas, E., Waern, M., Ostling, S., Guo, X. & Skoog, I. (2012). 37 years of body mass index and dementia: observations from the prospective population study of women in Gothenburg, Sweden. *J Alzheimers Dis, 28*, 163-171.

[181] Whitmer, R. A., Gunderson, E. P., Barrett-Connor, E., Quesenberry, C. P., Jr. & Yaffe, K. (2005). Obesity in middle age and future risk of dementia: a 27 year longitudinal population based study. *BMJ, 330*, 1360.

[182] O'Reilly, E. J., Wang, H., Weisskopf, M. G., Fitzgerald, K. C., Falcone, G., McCullough, M. L., Thun, M., et al. (2013). Premorbid body mass index and risk of amyotrophic lateral sclerosis. *Amyotroph Lateral Scler Frontotemporal Degener, 14*, 205-211.

[183] Bouteloup, C., Desport, J. C., Clavelou, P., Guy, N., Derumeaux-Burel, H., Ferrier, A. & Couratier, P. (2009). Hypermetabolism in ALS patients: an early and persistent phenomenon. *J Neurol, 256*, 1236-1242.

[184] World Health Organization (2012). *Diabetes Fact Sheet No.312.* Diabetes [cited July 30, 2014].

[185] Hu, G., Jousilahti, P., Bidel, S., Antikainen, R. & Tuomilehto, J. (2007). Type 2 diabetes and the risk of Parkinson's disease. *Diabetes Care, 30*, 842-847.

[186] Sims-Robinson, C., Kim, B., Rosko, A. & Feldman, E. L. (2010). How does diabetes accelerate Alzheimer disease pathology? *Nat Rev Neurol, 6*, 551-559.

[187] Rios, J. A., Cisternas, P., Arrese, M., Barja, S. & Inestrosa, N. C. (2014). Is Alzheimer's disease related to metabolic syndrome? A Wnt signaling conundrum. *Prog Neurobiol, 121*, 125-146.

[188] Lin, F., Lo, R. Y., Cole, D., Ducharme, S., Chen, D. G., Mapstone, M., Porsteinsson, A., et al. (2014). Longitudinal effects of metabolic syndrome on Alzheimer and vascular related brain pathology. *Dement Geriatr Cogn Dis Extra, 4*, 184-194.

[189] Zhang, P. & Tian, B. (2014). Metabolic syndrome: an important risk factor for Parkinson's disease. *Oxid Med Cell Longev, 2014*, 729194.

[190] Hu, G., Jousilahti, P., Nissinen, A., Antikainen, R., Kivipelto, M. & Tuomilehto, J. (2006). Body mass index and the risk of Parkinson disease. *Neurology, 67*, 1955-1959.

[191] Jawaid, A., Salamone, A. R., Strutt, A. M., Murthy, S. B., Wheaton, M., McDowell, E. J., Simpson, E., et al. (2010). ALS disease onset may occur later in patients with pre-morbid diabetes mellitus. *Eur J Neurol, 17*, 733-739.

[192] Iida, K. T., Shimano, H., Kawakami, Y., Sone, H., Toyoshima, H., Suzuki, S., Asano, T., et al. (2001). Insulin up-regulates tumor necrosis factor-alpha production in macrophages through an extracellular-regulated kinase-dependent pathway. *J Biol Chem, 276*, 32531-32537.

[193] Brundage, S. I., Kirilcuk, N. N., Lam, J. C., Spain, D. A. & Zautke, N. A. (2008). Insulin increases the release of proinflammatory mediators. *J Trauma, 65*, 367-372.

[194] Kawanishi, N., Yano, H., Yokogawa, Y. & Suzuki, K. (2010). Exercise training inhibits inflammation in adipose tissue via both suppression of macrophage infiltration and acceleration of phenotypic switching from M1 to M2 macrophages in high-fat-diet-induced obese mice. *Exerc Immunol Rev, 16*, 105-118.

[195] Gonzalez, A. S., Guerrero, D. B., Soto, M. B., Diaz, S. P., Martinez-Olmos, M. & Vidal, O. (2006). Metabolic syndrome, insulin resistance and the inflammation markers C-reactive protein and ferritin. *Eur J Clin Nutr, 60*, 802-809.

[196] Guldiken, S., Demir, M., Arikan, E., Turgut, B., Azcan, S., Gerenli, M. & Tugrul, A. (2007). The levels of circulating markers of atherosclerosis and inflammation in subjects with different degrees of body mass index:

Soluble CD40 ligand and high-sensitivity C-reactive protein. *Thromb Res, 119*, 79-84.

[197] Banks, W. A., Kastin, A. J. & Broadwell, R. D. (1995). Passage of cytokines across the blood-brain barrier. *Neuroimmunomodulation, 2*, 241-248.

[198] Drake, C., Boutin, H., Jones, M. S., Denes, A., McColl, B. W., Selvarajah, J. R., Hulme, S., et al. (2011). Brain inflammation is induced by co-morbidities and risk factors for stroke. *Brain Behav Immun, 25*, 1113-1122.

[199] Paul, D., Ge, S., Lemire, Y., Jellison, E. R., Serwanski, D. R., Ruddle, N. H. & Pachter, J. S. (2014). Cell-selective knockout and 3D confocal image analysis reveals separate roles for astrocyte-and endothelial-derived CCL2 in neuroinflammation. *J Neuroinflammation, 11*, 10.

[200] Zhang, X., Zhang, G., Zhang, H., Karin, M., Bai, H. & Cai, D. (2008). Hypothalamic IKKbeta/NF-kappaB and ER stress link overnutrition to energy imbalance and obesity. *Cell, 135*, 61-73.

[201] Thaler, J. P., Yi, C. X., Schur, E. A., Guyenet, S. J., Hwang, B. H., Dietrich, M. O., Zhao, X., et al. (2012). Obesity is associated with hypothalamic injury in rodents and humans. *J Clin Invest, 122*, 153-162.

[202] Tucsek, Z., Toth, P., Sosnowska, D., Gautam, T., Mitschelen, M., Koller, A., Szalai, G., et al. (2014). Obesity in aging exacerbates blood-brain barrier disruption, neuroinflammation, and oxidative stress in the mouse hippocampus: effects on expression of genes involved in beta-amyloid generation and Alzheimer's disease. *J Gerontol A Biol Sci Med Sci, 69*, 1212-1226.

[203] Dey, A., Hao, S., Erion, J. R., Wosiski-Kuhn, M. & Stranahan, A. M. (2014). Glucocorticoid sensitization of microglia in a genetic mouse model of obesity and diabetes. *J Neuroimmunol, 269*, 20-27.

[204] Parthsarathy, V. & Holscher, C. (2013). The type 2 diabetes drug liraglutide reduces chronic inflammation induced by irradiation in the mouse brain. *Eur J Pharmacol, 700*, 42-50.

[205] Little, J. P., Madeira, J. M. & Klegeris, A. (2012). The saturated fatty acid palmitate induces human monocytic cell toxicity toward neuronal cells: exploring a possible link between obesity-related metabolic impairments and neuroinflammation. *J Alzheimers Dis, 30 Suppl 2*, S179-183.

[206] Thirumangalakudi, L., Prakasam, A., Zhang, R., Bimonte-Nelson, H., Sambamurti, K., Kindy, M. S. & Bhat, N. R. (2008). High cholesterol-induced neuroinflammation and amyloid precursor protein processing

correlate with loss of working memory in mice. *J Neurochem, 106,* 475-485.

[207] Yang, F., Wang, Z., Zhang, J. H., Tang, J., Liu, X., Tan, L., Huang, Q. Y., et al. (2015). Receptor for advanced glycation end-product antagonist reduces blood-brain barrier damage after intracerebral hemorrhage. *Stroke, 46,* 1328-1336.

[208] Maisto, S. A., Galizio, M., Connors, G. J., Maheu, S. & McCarthy, A., *Drug Use and Abuse.* 1st Canadian Edition ed2013, Canada: Nelson Education.

[209] Keller, M. (1979). A historical overview of alcohol and alcoholism. *Cancer Res, 39,* 2822-2829.

[210] Marshall, S. A., McClain, J. A., Kelso, M. L., Hopkins, D. M., Pauly, J. R. & Nixon, K. (2013). Microglial activation is not equivalent to neuroinflammation in alcohol-induced neurodegeneration: The importance of microglia phenotype. *Neurobiol Dis, 54,* 239-251.

[211] Achur, R. N., Freeman, W. M. & Vrana, K. E. (2010). Circulating cytokines as biomarkers of alcohol abuse and alcoholism. *J Neuroimmune Pharmacol, 5,* 83-91.

[212] Crews, F. T., Zou, J. & Qin, L. (2011). Induction of innate immune genes in brain create the neurobiology of addiction. *Brain Behav Immun, 25 Suppl 1,* S4-S12.

[213] Pascual, M., Balino, P., Aragon, C. M. & Guerri, C. (2015). Cytokines and chemokines as biomarkers of ethanol-induced neuroinflammation and anxiety-related behavior: role of TLR4 and TLR2. *Neuropharmacology, 89,* 352-359.

[214] Yang, J. Y., Xue, X., Tian, H., Wang, X. X., Dong, Y. X., Wang, F., Zhao, Y. N., et al. (2014). Role of microglia in ethanol-induced neurodegenerative disease: Pathological and behavioral dysfunction at different developmental stages. *Pharmacol Ther, 144,* 321-337.

[215] Bajo, M., Varodayan, F. P., Madamba, S. G., Robert, A. J., Casal, L. M., Oleata, C. S., Siggins, G. R., et al. (2015). IL-1 interacts with ethanol effects on GABAergic transmission in the mouse central amygdala. *Front Pharmacol, 6,* 49.

[216] Hunt, W. A. (1983). The effect of ethanol on GABAergic transmission. *Neurosci Biobehav Rev, 7,* 87-95.

[217] Felderhoff-Mueser, U., Schmidt, O. I., Oberholzer, A., Buhrer, C. & Stahel, P. F. (2005). IL-18: a key player in neuroinflammation and neurodegeneration? *Trends Neurosci, 28,* 487-493.

[218] Checkoway, H., Powers, K., Smith-Weller, T., Franklin, G. M., Longstreth, W. T., Jr. & Swanson, P. D. (2002). Parkinson's disease risks associated with cigarette smoking, alcohol consumption, and caffeine intake. *Am J Epidemiol, 155,* 732-738.

[219] Barreto, G. E., Iarkov, A. & Moran, V. E. (2014). Beneficial effects of nicotine, cotinine and its metabolites as potential agents for Parkinson's disease. *Front Aging Neurosci, 6,* 340.

[220] Baez-Pagan, C. A., Delgado-Velez, M. & Lasalde-Dominicci, J. A. (2015). Activation of the Macrophage alpha7 Nicotinic Acetylcholine Receptor and Control of Inflammation. *J Neuroimmune Pharmacol, s11481.*

[221] Claassen, L., Papst, S., Reimers, K., Stukenborg-Colsman, C., Steinstraesser, L., Vogt, P. M., Kraft, T., et al. (2014). Inflammatory response to burn trauma: nicotine attenuates proinflammatory cytokine levels. *Eplasty, 14,* e46.

[222] Nizri, E., Irony-Tur-Sinai, M., Lory, O., Orr-Urtreger, A., Lavi, E. & Brenner, T. (2009). Activation of the cholinergic anti-inflammatory system by nicotine attenuates neuroinflammation via suppression of Th1 and Th17 responses. *J Immunol, 183,* 6681-6688.

[223] Albuquerque, E. X., Pereira, E. F., Alkondon, M. & Rogers, S. W. (2009). Mammalian nicotinic acetylcholine receptors: from structure to function. *Physiol Rev, 89,* 73-120.

[224] Rose, J. E., *The Clinical Management of Nicotine Dependence.* Transdermal Nicotine and Nasal Nicotine Administration as Smoking-Cessation Treatments, ed. J.A. Cocores 1991, New York: Springer-Verlag.

[225] Denissenko, M. F., Pao, A., Tang, M. & Pfeifer, G. P. (1996). Preferential formation of benzo[a]pyrene adducts at lung cancer mutational hotspots in P53. *Science, 274,* 430-432.

[226] Ambrose, J. A. & Barua, R. S. (2004). The pathophysiology of cigarette smoking and cardiovascular disease: an update. *J Am Coll Cardiol, 43,* 1731-1737.

[227] Scanlon, P. D., Connett, J. E., Waller, L. A., Altose, M. D., Bailey, W. C., Buist, A. S., Tashkin, D. P., et al. (2000). Smoking cessation and lung function in mild-to-moderate chronic obstructive pulmonary disease. The Lung Health Study. *Am J Respir Crit Care Med, 161,* 381-390.

[228] Kovalevich, J., Yen, W., Ozdemir, A. & Langford, D. (2015). Cocaine induces nuclear export and degradation of neuronal retinoid X receptor-

gamma via a TNF-alpha/JNK- mediated mechanism. *J Neuroimmune Pharmacol, 10*, 55-73.

[229] Kousik, S. M., Napier, T. C. & Carvey, P. M. (2012). The effects of psychostimulant drugs on blood brain barrier function and neuroinflammation. *Front Pharmacol, 3*, 121.

[230] Northrop, N. A. & Yamamoto, B. K. (2015). Methamphetamine effects on blood-brain barrier structure and function. *Front Neurosci, 9*, 69.

[231] Yang, L., Yao, H., Chen, X., Cai, Y., Callen, S. & Buch, S. (2015). Role of Sigma Receptor in Cocaine-Mediated Induction of Glial Fibrillary Acidic Protein: Implications for HAND. *Mol Neurobiol, s12035*.

[232] O'Shea, E., Urrutia, A., Green, A. R. & Colado, M. I. (2014). Current preclinical studies on neuroinflammation and changes in blood-brain barrier integrity by MDMA and methamphetamine. *Neuropharmacology, 87*, 125-134.

[233] van de Haar, H. J., Burgmans, S., Hofman, P. A., Verhey, F. R., Jansen, J. F. & Backes, W. H. (2015). Blood-brain barrier impairment in dementia: current and future in vivo assessments. *Neurosci Biobehav Rev, 49*, 71-81.

[234] Goldstein, A., *Addiction: From Biology to Drug Policy.* 2nd ed2001, USA: Oxford University Press.

[235] Rock, R. B., Hu, S., Sheng, W. S. & Peterson, P. K. (2006). Morphine stimulates CCL2 production by human neurons. *J Neuroinflammation, 3*, 32.

[236] Deshmane, S. L., Kremlev, S., Amini, S. & Sawaya, B. E. (2009). Monocyte chemoattractant protein-1 (MCP-1): an overview. *J Interferon Cytokine Res, 29*, 313-326.

[237] Neri, M., Panata, L., Bacci, M., Fiore, C., Riezzo, I., Turillazzi, E. & Fineschi, V. (2013). Cytokines, chaperones and neuroinflammatory responses in heroin-related death: what can we learn from different patterns of cellular expression? *Int J Mol Sci, 14*, 19831-19845.

[238] Dale, E., Bang-Andersen, B. & Sánchez, C. (2015). Emerging mechanisms and treatments for depression beyond SSRIs and SNRIs. *Biochem Pharmacol, 95*, 81-97.

[239] Koschnitzky, J. E., Quinlan, K. A., Lukas, T. J., Kajtaz, E., Kocevar, E. J., Mayers, W. F., Siddique, T., et al. (2014). Effect of fluoxetine on disease progression in a mouse model of ALS. *J Neurophysiol, 111*, 2164-2176.

[240] Fonseka, T. M., McIntyre, R. S., Soczynska, J. K. & Kennedy, S. H. (2015). Novel investigational drugs targeting IL-6 signaling for the treatment of depression. *Expert Opin Investig Drugs*, *24*, 459-475.

[241] O'Sullivan, J., Ryan, K., Harkin, A. & Connor, T. (2010). Noradrenaline reuptake inhibitors inhibit expression of chemokines IP-10 and RANTES and cell adhesion molecules VCAM-1 and ICAM-1 in the CNS following a systemic inflammatory challenge. *J Neuroimmunol*, *220*, 34-42.

[242] Schmitt, J. A., Wingen, M., Ramaekers, J. G., Evers, E. A. & Riedel, W. J. (2006). Serotonin and human cognitive performance. *Curr Pharm Des*, *12*, 2473-2486.

[243] National Collaborating Centre for Mental Health. (2010), *Depression : the treatment and management of depression in adults*. Updated ed. ed2010, London: British Psychological Society and the Royal College of Psychiatrists.

[244] Hwang, J., Zheng, L. T., Ock, J., Lee, M. G., Kim, S. H., Lee, H. W., Lee, W. H., et al. (2008). Inhibition of glial inflammatory activation and neurotoxicity by tricyclic antidepressants. *Neuropharmacology*, *55*, 826-834.

[245] Lee, Y. H., Kim, S. H., Kim, Y., Lim, Y., Ha, K. & Shin, S. Y. (2012). Inhibitory effect of the antidepressant imipramine on NF-κB-dependent CXCL1 expression in TNFα-exposed astrocytes. *Int Immunopharmacol*, *12*, 547-555.

[246] Cassano, G. B., Heinze, G., Lôo, H., Mendlewicz, J. & Sousa, M. P. (1996). A double-blind comparison of tianeptine, imipramine and placebo in the treatment of major depressive episodes. *Eur Psychiatry*, *11*, 254-259.

[247] Hannestad, J., DellaGioia, N. & Bloch, M. (2011). The effect of antidepressant medication treatment on serum levels of inflammatory cytokines: a meta-analysis. *Neuropsychopharmacology*, *36*, 2452-2459.

[248] Horowitz, M. A., Wertz, J., Zhu, D., Cattaneo, A., Musaelyan, K., Nikkheslat, N., Thuret, S., et al. (2015). Antidepressant compounds can be both pro- and anti-inflammatory in human hippocampal cells. *Int J Neuropsychopharmacol*, *18*, 1-9.

[249] Tynan, R. J., Weidenhofer, J., Hinwood, M., Cairns, M. J., Day, T. A. & Walker, F. R. (2012). A comparative examination of the anti-inflammatory effects of SSRI and SNRI antidepressants on LPS stimulated microglia. *Brain Behav Immun*, *26*, 469-479.

[250] Troib, A. & Azab, A. N. (2015). Effects of psychotropic drugs on Nuclear Factor kappa B. *Eur Rev Med Pharmacol Sci, 19*, 1198-1208.

[251] Porterfield, V. M., Zimomra, Z. R., Caldwell, E. A., Camp, R. M., Gabella, K. M. & Johnson, J. D. (2011). Rat strain differences in restraint stress-induced brain cytokines. *Neuroscience, 188*, 48-54.

[252] Peters, V. A., Joesting, J. J. & Freund, G. G. (2013). IL-1 receptor 2 (IL-1R2) and its role in immune regulation. *Brain Behav Immun, 32*, 1-8.

[253] Smith, D., Dempster, C., Glanville, J., Freemantle, N. & Anderson, I. (2002). Efficacy and tolerability of venlafaxine compared with selective serotonin reuptake inhibitors and other antidepressants: a meta-analysis. *Br J Psychiatry, 180*, 396-404.

[254] Trudler, D., Weinreb, O., Mandel, S. A., Youdim, M. B. & Frenkel, D. (2014). DJ-1 deficiency triggers microglia sensitivity to dopamine toward a pro-inflammatory phenotype that is attenuated by rasagiline. *J Neurochem, 129*, 434-447.

[255] Al-Nuaimi, S. K., Mackenzie, E. M. & Baker, G. B. (2012). Monoamine oxidase inhibitors and neuroprotection: a review. *Am J Ther, 19*, 436-448.

[256] Panarsky, R., Luques, L. & Weinstock, M. (2012). Anti-inflammatory effects of ladostigil and its metabolites in aged rat brain and in microglial cells. *J Neuroimmune Pharmacol, 7*, 488-498.

[257] Carradori, S. & Petzer, J. P. (2015). Novel monoamine oxidase inhibitors: a patent review (2012 - 2014). *Expert Opin Ther Pat, 25*, 91-110.

[258] Coyle, C. M. & Laws, K. R. (2015). The use of ketamine as an antidepressant: a systematic review and meta-analysis. *Hum Psychopharmacol, 30*, 152-163.

[259] Price, D. L., Rockenstein, E., Ubhi, K., Van, P., MacLean-Lewis, N., Askay, D., Cartier, A., et al. (2010). Alterations in mGluR5 Expression and Signaling in Lewy Body Disease and in Transgenic Models of Alpha-Synucleinopathy - Implications for Excitotoxicity. *Plos One, 5*, 1-16.

[260] Parsons, M. P. & Raymond, L. A. (2014). Extrasynaptic NMDA Receptor Involvement in Central Nervous System Disorders. *Neuron, 82*, 279-293.

[261] Meng, C., Liu, Z., Liu, G. L., Fu, L. S., Zhang, M., Zhang, Z., Xia, H. M., et al. (2015). Ketamine promotes inflammation through increasing TLR4 expression in RAW264.7 cells. *J Huazhong Univ Sci Technolog Med Sci, 35*, 419-425.

[262] Tan, Y., Wang, Q., She, Y., Bi, X. & Zhao, B. (2015). Ketamine reduces LPS-induced HMGB1 via activation of the Nrf2/HO-1 pathway and NF-κB suppression. *J Trauma Acute Care Surg, 78*, 784-792.

[263] Kang, M. G., Byun, K., Kim, J. H., Park, N. H., Heinsen, H., Ravid, R., Steinbusch, H. W., et al. (2015). Proteogenomics of the human hippocampus: The road ahead. *Biochim Biophys Acta, 1854*, 788-797.

[264] Buchanan, C. R., Pettit, L. D., Storkey, A. J., Abrahams, S. & Bastin, M. E. (2015). Reduced structural connectivity within a prefrontal-motor-subcortical network in amyotrophic lateral sclerosis. *J Magn Reson Imaging, 41*, 1342-1352.

[265] Wilson, R. S., Barnes, L. L., Bennett, D. A., Li, Y., Bienias, J. L., de Leon, C. F. M. & Evans, D. A. (2005). Proneness to psychological distress and risk of Alzheimer disease in a biracial community. *Neurology, 64*, 380-382.

[266] Miller, A. H., Maletic, V. & Raison, C. L. (2009). Inflammation and Its Discontents: The Role of Cytokines in the Pathophysiology of Major Depression. *Biol Psychiatry, 65*, 732-741.

[267] Amieva, H., Le Goff, M., Millet, X., Orgogozo, J. M., Peres, K., Barberger-Gateau, P., Jacqmin-Gadda, H., et al. (2008). Prodromal Alzheimer's Disease: Successive Emergence of the Clinical Symptoms. *Ann Neurol, 64*, 492-498.

[268] Perez Nievas, B. G., Hammerschmidt, T., Kummer, M. P., Terwel, D., Leza, J. C. & Heneka, M. T. (2011). Restraint stress increases neuroinflammation independently of amyloid β levels in amyloid precursor protein/PS1 transgenic mice. *J Neurochem, 116*, 43-52.

[269] Leonard, B. E. & Myint, A. (2006). Changes in the immune system in depression and dementia: causal or coincidental effects? *Dialogues Clin Neurosci, 8*, 163-174.

[270] Perry, V. H. & Teeling, J. (2013). Microglia and macrophages of the central nervous system: the contribution of microglia priming and systemic inflammation to chronic neurodegeneration. *Semin Immunopathol, 35*, 601-612.

[271] Craig, D., Mirakhur, A., Hart, D. J., McIlroy, S. P. & Passmore, A. P. (2005). A cross-sectional study of neuropsychiatric symptoms in 435 patients with Alzheimer's disease. *Am J Geriatr Psychiatry, 13*, 460-468.

[272] Wuwongse, S., Chang, R. C.-C. & Law, A. C. K. (2010). The putative neurodegenerative links between depression and Alzheimer's disease. *Prog Neurobiol, 91*, 362-375.

[273] Liu, W. N., Sheng, H., Xu, Y. J., Liu, Y., Lu, J. Q. & Ni, X. (2013). Swimming exercise ameliorates depression-like behavior in chronically stressed rats: Relevant to proinflammatory cytokines and IDO activation. *Behav Brain Res*, *242*, 110-116.

[274] Dobos, N., Korf, J., Luiten, P. G. M. & Eisel, U. L. M. (2010). Neuroinflammation in Alzheimer's Disease and Major Depression. *Biol Psychiatry*, *67*, 503-504.

[275] O'Connor, J. C., Andre, C., Wang, Y. X., Lawson, M. A., Szegedi, S. S., Lestage, J., Castanon, N., et al. (2009). Interferon-gamma and Tumor Necrosis Factor-alpha Mediate the Upregulation of Indoleamine 2,3-Dioxygenase and the Induction of Depressive-Like Behavior in Mice in Response to Bacillus Calmette-Guerin. *J Neurosci*, *29*, 4200-4209.

[276] Johnson, R. W., Freund, G. G., Kelley, K. W., O'Connor, J. C. & Dantzer, R. (2008). From inflammation to sickness and depression: when the immune system subjugates the brain. *Nat Rev Neurosci*, *9*, 46-56.

[277] Raison, C. L., Capuron, L. & Miller, A. H. (2006). Cytokines sing the blues: inflammation and the pathogenesis of depression. *Trends Immunol*, *27*, 24-31.

[278] Frodl, T. & O'Keane, V. (2013). How does the brain deal with cumulative stress? A review with focus on developmental stress, HPA axis function and hippocampal structure in humans. *Neurobiol Dis*, *52*, 24-37.

[279] Hanstein, R., Lu, A., Wurst, W., Holsboer, F., Deussing, J. M., Clement, A. B. & Behl, C. (2008). Transgenic overexpression of corticotropin releasing hormone provides partial protection against neurodegeneration in an in vivo model of acute excitotoxic stress. *Neuroscience*, *156*, 712-721.

In: Neuroinflammation in Disease
Editor: Rebecca K. Dawson

ISBN: 978-1-63483-389-9
© 2015 Nova Science Publishers, Inc.

Chapter II

Therapeutic Effects of Estrogen Receptor Agonists in Inhibition of Neuroinflammation in Different Neurological Disorders

***Mrinmay Chakrabarti and Swapan K. Ray**[*]
Department of Pathology, Microbiology, and Immunology,
University of South Carolina School of Medicine,
Columbia, South Carolina, US

Abstract

There are multiple connections between the central nervous system (CNS) and the immune system so as to regulate the innate immune responses for normal neurological functions in humans. Microglial cells play the most crucial role against wound or microbial infection and stimulate an array of secondary responses through astrocyte activation and recruitment of peripheral immune cells into the CNS. Estrogen receptor agonists (ERAs) can modulate

[*] Corresponding author: Swapan K. Ray, PhD, Department of Pathology, Microbiology, and Immunology, University of South Carolina School of Medicine, Building 2, Room C11, 6439 Garners Ferry Road, Columbia, SC 29209, USA. Phone: 803-216-3420; Fax: 803-216-3428; E-mail: swapan.ray@uscmed.sc.edu.

the activity of many cell types involved in the immune response in the CNS. Recent studies confirmed that ERAs could modulate different inflammatory processes in animal models of human CNS diseases such as multiple sclerosis (MS), epilepsy, Parkinson's disease (PD), Alzheimer disease (AD), and spinal cord injury (SCI). Recent studies demonstrated that ERAs can control activation of microglia, migration of blood-derived monocytes to the infected area, and inhibition of expression of pro-inflammatory cytokines (IL-1β and TNF-α) in the CNS. Neuroprotective effects of ERAs are mainly mediated by estrogen receptor alpha (ERα) and ER beta (ERβ), which are a member of the nuclear hormone family of intracellular receptors. ERs are expressed in various cell types of the immune system, including macrophages, microglia, and T cells. The exact mechanisms of modulation of different neuroinflammatory pathways in the CNS are not completely known. Research on ERAs and different CNS disorders still remains in its early stage but several studies have indicated promising therapeutic effects of ERAs in delaying the onset neuroinflammation and thus symptomatic recovery in some CNS disorders. This book chapter will highlight some recent developments on mechanisms of action and therapeutic effects of ERAs in prevention of neurodegeneration and neuroinflammation in different CNS disorders.

Introduction

Numerous investigations support the prominent role of inflammation in the pathogenesis and advancement of neurodegenerative disorders such as multiple sclerosis (MS), Alzheimer's disease (AD), and Parkinson's disease (PD). Microglial cells, the resident immune cells in the brain, are mainly responsible in promoting inflammatory response against external stimuli. Activated microglia neutralizes foreign bodies or cell debris by phagocytosis (engulfing foreign bodies) and also can release inflammatory molecules to facilitate the inflammatory response. Conversely, disproportionate activation of microglial cells may damage nearby host cells and also develop some neuronal inflammatory diseases due high level secretion of cytokines and other inflammatory molecules such as reactive oxygen species (ROS), nitric oxide (NO), cyclooxygenase-2 (COX-2), tumor necrosis factor-α (TNF-α), and interleukin-1β (IL-1β) in the CNS or cerebrospinal fluid [Ishihara et al. 2015]. A significant population of activated microglial cells have been observed in the histopathological sites during the pathogenesis of AD, PD, ischemia–

reperfusion injury, trauma, epilepsy, depression, and schizophrenia, suggesting that microglia-mediated inflammatory responses may be a mechanism in many neurodegenerative diseases [Hickman et al. 2008; Marinova-Mutafchieva et al. 2009; Wang et al. 2011; Najjar et al. 2013; Xanthos and Sandkuhler, 2014]. Therefore, understanding the molecular mechanisms of microglia activation and regulation can be beneficial for the development new therapeutic strategies against different neurodegenerative disorders that are associated with a common neuroinflammatory progression.

A large number of preclinical and basic neurobiological investigations reported significant neuroprotective potential of estrogen (EST) and estrogen receptor agonists (ERAs) against many neurodegenerative diseases [Vegeto et al. 2008; Chakrabarti et al. 2014a, 2014b]. Treatment with EST and ERAs block inflammatory cytokine production and NO generation induced by lipopolysaccharide (LPS) in microglia [Bruce-Keller et al. 2000; Vegeto et al. 2001; Xing et al. 2008]. The anti-inflammatory responses of EST and ERAs are mediated via the classical estrogen receptor alpha (ERα) and ER beta (ERβ) so as to suppress the transcriptional activity of the key pro-inflammatory signaling molecule nuclear factor-kappa B (NF-κB) p65 [Ghisletti et al. 2005]. Some in vivo models of the CNS diseases also demonstrated anti-inflammatory roles of EST via ER-dependent pathway [Vegeto et al. 2003; Brown et al. 2010]. Although the neuroprotective and anti-inflammatory potential of EST and ERAs in the CNS are well recognizable in animal models of neurodegenerative diseases, their clinical use is still controversial because of the secondary effects in reproductive organs and potential risk of cancer development. Obviously, alternative compounds of EST with similar mode of action should be developed for different CNS disorders with a better safety profile than EST. The aim of this chapter is to discuss the contemporary knowledge on ERA action in neurodegenerative pathological conditions and to support the idea that ERAs may delay the commencement and progression of neurodegeneration with lower side effects in surrounding tissues.

Mechanisms of Inhibition of Neuroinflammation by EST and ERAs

EST and ERAs are known to act via the activation of the endogenous ERα and ERβ (Figure 1). Both receptors can be activated via direct genomic pathway or indirect non-genomic pathway in neural cells [Maggi et al. 2004]. The ER antagonist ICI 182780 has been observed to block the effect of the hormonal action EST in microglia [Brown et al. 2008]. Although ERβ is extensively expressed in most of cells in the CNS, studies suggest that it does not contribute to the protective effect of EST in inflammatory brain diseases [Mitra et al. 2003]. Several in vivo studies with ER-deficient mice demonstrated the selective requirement of ERα not ERβ in the neuroprotective and anti-inflammatory action of EST during neuropathological conditions [Vegeto et al. 2003; Polanczyk et al. 2005]. On the contrary, Harris and coworkers reported tissue and signal specific involvement of both ERα and ERβ in controlling the inflammation [Harris et al. 2003]. Whether ERα or ERβ, or both ERs induce cell specific responses for prevention of inflammatory process is still controversial and more studies are needed to confirm it.

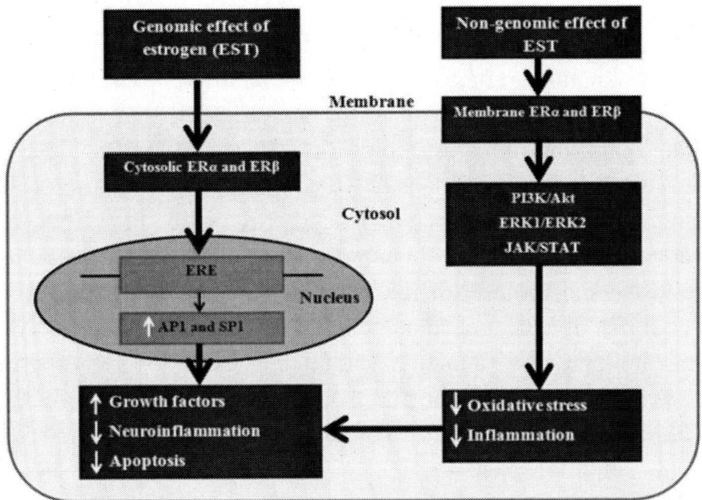

Figure 1. EST and ERA signaling is mediated by both genomic and non-genomic mechanisms. In genomic mechanism, ERs act as ligand-activated transcription factors, activating or repressing target genes. ERs are located as monomers and also as protein complexes in the cell cytosol. EST binding induces their dissociation from this complex and ER dimerization. ER dimers then enter into the nucleus and bind directly to estrogen response elements (ERE) at the promoters of the target genes (AP1 and SP1). EST and ERAs also regulate different physiological processes in a ligand independent manner (non-genomic pathway) through activation of different intracellular kinases. This non-genomic pathway involves activation of ERs and G-protein-coupled ER located at cell membrane resulting in stimulation of different kinases such as PI3K/Akt, ERK1/ERK2, and JAK/STAT for suppression of oxidative stress and inflammation.

ERAs and selective estrogen receptor modulators (SERMs) without feminizing effects of EST could be the ideal alternatives to enhance cognitive function during different neuropathological conditions [Zhao et al. 2005]. ERs are candidate targets for neuroprotective therapies based on EST actions [DonCarlos et al. 2009]. Several cell culture and animal studies reported beneficial and neuroprotective roles of SERMs such as tamoxifen, raloxifene, or genistein [Zhao et al. 2005, Azcoitia et al. 2006; Kokiko et al. 2006]. The neuroprotective action of EST and ERAs in the brain is generally facilitated by their binding to classical nuclear ERs (ERα and ERβ) (Figure 1). Both ERs belong to the steroid and thyroid hormone receptor superfamily and acts as ligand inducible transcription factors [Nilsson et al. 2001]. Upon activation, ERs can form dimers, interact with the estrogen responsive elements (ERE) and recruit many transcriptional co-factors to the regulatory regions of the specific genes. Furthermore, the activated ERs help other transcription factors to bind and stabilize the specific ERE in the target DNA and recruit other specific co-repressors and co-activators that eventually stimulate transcriptional machinery [DonCarlos et al. 2009]. Therapeutic strategy with SERMs against many neurodisorders is advantageous because they mimic EST action in some brain regions but showed anti-estrogenic effects in other brain regions or peripheral tissues [DonCarlos et al. 2009].

Neuroprotective Roles of EST and ERAs in Multiple Sclerosis

Multiple sclerosis (MS) is a major neurological disorder that occurs due to invasion of immune cells into the CNS resulting in destruction of myelin, death of oligodendrocytes, axon degeneration, and neuronal damage [Vegeto et al. 2008]. Although, MS occurs more frequently in women than in men, it affects men with quicker progression [Wynn et al. 1990]. The effects of EST and ERAs on immune system are thought to be biphasic: low doses of EST stimulate pro-inflammatory Th1 responses and enhance cell-mediated immunity, but at higher doses they promote anti-inflammatory Th2 responses [Buyon, 1998]. Few recent studies suggested that low oral doses of EST significantly decreased the acuteness of *experimental autoimmune encephalomyelitis* (EAE, an animal model of MS) with suppression of chemokines and pro-inflammatory Th1 cytokines (IL-1, IL-6, IFN-γ, and TNF-α), and induced expression of anti-inflammatory Th2 cytokines (IL-4, IL-5, and TGF-β) [Vegeto et al. 2008]. A similar animal study reported that EST could protect mice from EAE by blocking the recruitment of macrophages and T cells into the CNS [Subramanian et al. 2003]. Treatment with an ERα specific agonist can inhibit acute EAE pathogenesis through induction of EST mediated neuroprotective pathways [Elloso et al. 2005; Morales et al. 2006].

EST mediated neuroprotective activity in MS or EAE is generally carried out through inhibition of neutrophils, monocytes, macrophages, and different subtypes of T cells. EST and ERAs are capable of altering the T cell population towards a Th2 phenotype and also induce a subpopulation of T regulatory (Treg) cells [Vegeto et al. 2008]. Alternatively, the neuroprotective potential of ERAs on MS and EAE may not involve ERα signaling in blood-derived inflammatory cells, but depends on ERα expressed in the CNS resident microglia or endothelial cells [Garidou et al. 2004]. Thus, more studies are needed to confirm that the neuroprotective effects of EST and ERAs on MS and EAE are mediated through ERα signaling mechanisms in inflammatory cells, including macrophages and T cells.

Neuroprotective Roles of EST and ERAs in Alzheimer's Disease

Randomized clinical trials indicated the enhanced risk of Alzheimer's disease (AD) and dementia following EST therapy in women participating at the Women Health Initiative Study [Rapp et al. 2003; Espeland et al. 2004]. On the contrary, many epidemiological studies indicated a reverse correlation between EST therapy and occurrence of AD [Nilsson and Gustafsson, 2011]. Many well-controlled investigations were performed in experimental animal models that supported the protective roles of EST against neuronal damage. EST deficient aromatase gene knockout mice have been observed an increase in hippocampal neuronal loss following neurotoxin insult when compared with wild-type mice [Azcoitia et al. 2001]. Similarly, brain EST levels and aromatase expression were drastically decreased in the brains of women diagnosed with AD [Yue et al. 2005]. Many similar studies described that EST deficiency in brain could be a risk factor for generation of AD pathology [Vest and Pike, 2013].

Several experimental evidences suggest that EST and ERAs protect against amyloid beta (Aβ) neurotoxicity. EST enhances production of *amyloid precursor protein (APP)* in neuronal cells and suppresses Aβ peptide generation by scavenging mechanism [Xu et al. 1998]. A triple transgenic mouse model of AD was used to determine the efficacy of monotherapy and combination therapy with EST and progesterone on various pathological conditions [Carroll et al. 2007]. Drastic accumulation of Aβ deteriorated memory performance that was observed following ovariectomy (ovary removal surgery). But, chronic EST therapy could prevent the AD pathological symptoms. Following a combination treatment with EST and progesterone, progesterone antagonized the therapeutic effects of EST on Aβ accumulation without affecting behavioral outcomes. But progesterone considerably lessened tau hyperphosphorylation when treated alone or in combination with EST [Carroll et al. 2007]. Collectively, all these investigations indicated that EST insufficiency in brain could induce AD pathological conditions and symptoms, and EST and ERA treatment could inhibit the progression of AD.

Several studies were conducted to demonstrate the ability of EST in controlling inflammatory cells in brain reactivity in details [Vegeto et al. 2001; Vegeto et al. 2003; Vegeto et al. 2006]. The numbers of reactive microglia associated plaques were enhanced with time, indicating that the neuroinflammatory process was actually going on simultaneously with the disease progression. Ovariectomy enhanced activation of microglial cells encircling Aβ plaques and EST therapy blocked this neuroinflammatory process. Similarly, EST treatment significantly inhibited expression of inflammatory genes like macrophage inflammatory protein-2 (MIP-2), macrophage chemoattractant protein-1 (MCP-1), and TNF-α stimulated by *lipopolysaccharide* (*LPS*) administration in the cerebral ventricles [Vegeto et al. 2001]. Thus, these studies clearly suggest the important anti-inflammatory role of EST to prevent pathogenesis of AD through direct modulation of resident microglia in the CNS. In addition to the microgial regulation, EST also exhibited prominent protective effects in neurons, neural stem cells, astroglial cells, and endothelial cells through its anti-apoptotic, neurotrophic, and cell proliferative actions in the CNS [Maggi et al. 2004; Pozzi et al. 2006].

Neuroprotective Roles of EST and ERAs in Parkinson's Disease

Parkinson's disease (PD) is characterized by selective and progressive loss of dopamine (DA) producing neuronal cell bodies in substantia nigra resulting in an imbalance in the control of movement [Bourque et al. 2012]. Several epidemiological investigations suggest that the occurrence of PD is higher in men than in women [Bourque et al. 2012]. The beneficial effect of EST treatment on PD has been documented in many clinical reports confirming the role of endogenous and exogenous EST in modulating PD symptoms [Kompoliti et al. 2000; Tolson et al. 2002]. Additionally, EST replacement therapy recovers motor disability in PD post-menopausal women with motor instabilities [Tsang et al. 2000] and lessens symptom severity in women with early stage PD not treating with L-Dopa [Saunders-Pullman et al. 1999]. An enhanced risk of dementia existed in overiectomy women and the effect might be age-dependent [Rocca et al. 2007]. Thus, above studies clearly indicated the important beneficial role of EST in preventing the pathogenesis of PD.

Many animal studies explored the sensitivity of dopaminergic neurons to EST and observed that EST promoted DA synthesis, release, and differentiation of dopaminergic neurons [Morissette et al. 1993; McDermott et al. 1994]. In some earlier studies, the neurotoxin 1-methyl-4-phenyl-1,2,3,6-tetrahydropyridine (MPTP) was observed to induce more DA exhaustion in male than female mice [Dluzen et al. 1996] and EST therapy could block the decrease in DA level with activation of glia in the striatum of animals [Morale et al. 2006; Tripanichkul et al. 2006]. A dependable mouse model of PD was invented using MPTP [Jackson-Lewis and Przedborski, 2007]. Collectively, all the pilot clinical studies indicated promising outcomes from EST treatment considering hormone therapy safety and effectiveness in PD [Liu and Dluzen, 2007]. Although, the exact mechanism of EST-microglia signaling pathway in PD is still missing, several studies have confirmed that EST can avert microglia activation induced by neurotoxic insults [Vegeto et al. 2008]. Thus, it is believed that EST and ERAs may provide beneficial outcome on neurons, astrocytes, and microglia, and represent very possible pharmacological agents for preventing PD pathogenesis.

Neuroprotective Roles of EST and ERAs in Epilepsy

Several earlier and recent studies demonstrated that EST could prevent neuronal death from diverse neurotoxic insults such as glutamate excitotoxicity [Hilton et al. 2006], ischemia [Guo et al. 2010], kainic acid (KA)-induced toxicity [Hoffman et al. 2006], etc. However, EST is not recommended for the treatment of epilepsy to prevent seizure-induced cell death because it brings down the seizure threshold resulting in acceleration of seizures [Reddy, 2009]. Its use as hormone replacement therapy is linked with several damaging consequences such as increased risk of endometrial adenocarcinoma [Gambrell et al. 1983] and proliferation of breast epithelium [Russo and Irma, 2006]. Recently some selective EST receptor modulators (SERMs) have been developed those can overcome the limitations of EST for the treatment different diseases including neurological disorders (Table 1). These SERMs have shown diverse effect in the CNS by acting as ERAs in bone, cardiovascular system and brain, and as an antagonist in uterus and breast [Ibrahim and Hortobagyi, 1999], and thus have emerged as a replacement for providing neuroprotection [Arevalo et al. 2011]. Raloxifene (RLX) has been shown to prevent KA induced neurotoxicity in the hippocampus and it is approved for the treatment of osteoporosis [Ciriza et al. 2004]. Also, RLX lowered the pathogenesis of epilepsy with less number of seizures and delayed the latency of seizures after pilocarpine-induced status epilepticus (SE) in rats [Scharfman et al. 2009].

Table 1. SERMs and their action in neurological and other diseases

Name	Applications	Mode of action
Tamoxifen	Metastatic breast cancer, McCune-Albright syndrome, infertility, gynecomastia, bipolar disorder, angiogenesis and cancer, and control of gene expression	Antagonist at breast tissues, agonist at uterus and bone
Raloxifene	Invasive breast cancer, vertebral fractures, and osteoporosis	Antagonist at breast and uterus, agonist at bone
Lasofoxifene	Osteoporosis, vaginal atrophy, ER-positive breast cancer, coronary heart disease, and stroke	Antagonist at breast and uterus, agonist at the bone
Ospemifene	Dyspareunia and vaginal atrophy	Antagonist at breast and uterus, agonist at the bone
Clomifene	Anovulation or oligoovulation	Antagonist of estrogen receptors in the hypothalamus
Toremifene	Advanced metastatic breast cancer and prostatic intraepithelial neoplasia	Blocks the effects of estrogen in the breast tissue
Ormeloxifene	Contraceptive, menorrhagia, mastalgia, and fibroadenoma	Antagonist at breast and uterus, agonist at bone
Femarelle	Treatment of menopause and promotion osteoblast activity	Agonist at brain and bone

The transforming growth factor-beta (TGF-β) is a multifunctional peptide growth factor involved in the regulation of proliferation, differentiation, and survival and also it acts as an important mediator in the pathophysiology of inflammation and tissue repair [Kim et al. 2002]. Ectopic overexpression of TGF-β3 has been observed to reduce KA-induced seizures and neuronal damage significantly in rat models of epilepsy [Kim et al. 2002]. Hence, TGF-β signaling plays a significant role in protective mechanisms against KA-induced epileptogenesis and secondary tissue damage in brain. Ovariectomy is the most frequently used in vivo model to investigate the potential of EST and ERAs in epilepsy pathology [Schauwecker et al. 2009] as it affects physiological levels of EST and excludes all ovarian secretions [Schauwecker et al. 2009]. The industrial chemical 4-vinylcyclohexene diepoxide (VCD) selectively kills the small primordial and primary ovarian follicles leading to a gradual decline in reproductive activity and is considered to model menopause in rodents [Mayer et al. 2002].

Conclusion

The recent evidences clearly indicate the significant roles of EST and ERAs in modulating anti-inflammatory responses in the CNS to provide neuroprotection against diverse neurotoxic agents. Several in vivo studies suggested that cell specificity, receptor selectivity, and hormonal dose are the most crucial features for the effectiveness of EST and ERAs to regulate microglia and brain inflammation. Microglia activation associated with neurodegenerative processes may also have advantageous effects, as microglia cells generate trophic and survival factors that help to remove toxic materials through phagocytosis. Additional investigation is required to effectively establish the neuroprotective potency of available SERMs and other ERAs in different neurological disorders. Finally, future research may lead to development of the most suitable and effective estrogenic agent for using as therapy in different neuroinflammatory diseases.

Acknowledgments

This work was supported in part by the SC SCIRF-2015-I-01 and USC SOM RDF grants.

References

Arevalo, MA; Santos-Galindo, M; Lagunas, N; Azcoitia, I; Garcia-Segura, LM. Selective oestrogen receptor modulators as brain therapeutic agents. *J Mol Endocrinol*, 2011, 46, 1-9.

Azcoitia, I; Sierra, A; Garcia-Segura, LM. Neuroprotective effects of estradiol in the adult rat hippocampus: interaction with insulin-like growth factor-I signalling. *J Neurosci Res*, 1999, 58, 815-822.

Azcoitia, I; Sierra, A; Veiga, S; Honda, S; Harada, N; Garcia-Segura, LM. Brain aromatase is neuroprotective. *J Neurobiol*, 2001, 47, 318-329.

Bourque, M; Dluzen, DE; Di, Paolo T. Signaling pathways mediating the neuroprotective effects of sex steroids and SERMs in Parkinson's disease. *Front Neuroendocrinol*, 2012, 33, 169-178.

Brown, CM; Choi, E; Xu, Q; Vitek, MP; Colton, CA. The APOE4 genotype alters the response of microglia and macrophages to 17beta-estradiol. *Neurobiol Aging*, 2008, 29, 1783-1794.

Brown, CM; Mulcahey, TA; Filipek, NC; Wise, PM. Production of proinflammatory cytokines and chemokines during neuroinflammation: novel roles for estrogen receptors alpha and beta. *Endocrinology*, 2010, 151, 4916-4925.

Bruce-Keller, AJ; Keeling, JL; Keller, JN; Huang, FF; Camondola, S; Mattson, MP. Antiinflammatory effects of estrogen on microglial activation. *Endocrinology*, 2000, 141, 3646-3656.

Buyon, JP. The effects of pregnancy on autoimmune diseases. *J Leukoc Biol*, 1998, 63, 281-287.

Carroll, JC; Rosario, ER; Chang, L; Stanczyk, FZ; Oddo, S; LaFerla, FM; Pike, CJ. Progesterone and estrogen regulate Alzheimer-like neuropathology in female 3xTg-AD mice. *J Neurosci*, 2007, 27, 13357-13365.

Chakrabarti, M; Banik, NL; Ray, SK. miR-7-1 potentiated estrogen receptor agonists for functional neuroprotection in VSC4.1 motoneurons. *Neuroscience*, 2014b, 256, 322-33.

Chakrabarti, M; Haque, A; Banik, NL; Nagarkatti, P; Nagarkatti, M; Ray, SK. Estrogen receptor agonists for attenuation of neuroinflammation and neurodegeneration. *Brain Res Bull*, 2014a, 109, 22-31.

Ciriza, I; Carrero, P; Azcoitia, I; Lundeen, SG; Garcia-Segura, LM. Selective oestrogen receptor modulators protect hippocampal neurones from kainic acid excitotoxicity: differences with the effect of estradiol. *J Neurobiol*, 2004, 61, 209-221.

Dluzen, DE; McDermott, JL; Liu, B. Estrogen as a neuroprotectant against MPTP-induced neurotoxicity in C57/BL mice. *Neurotoxicol Teratol*, 1996, 18, 603-606.

DonCarlos, LL; Azcoitia, I; Garcia-Segura, LM. Neuroprotective actions of selective estrogen receptor modulators. *Psychoneuroendocrinology*, 2009, 34 Suppl 1, S113-22.

Elloso, MM; Phiel, K; Henderson, RA; Harris, HA; Adelman, SJ. Suppression of experimental autoimmune encephalomyelitis using estrogen receptor-selective ligands. *J Endocrinol*, 2005, 185, 243-252.

Espeland, MA; Rapp, SR; Shumaker, SA; Brunner, R; Manson, JE; Sherwin, BB; Hsia, J; Margolis, KL; Hogan, PE; Wallace, R; Dailey, M; Freeman, R; Hays, J. Women's health initiative memory study. Conjugated equine estrogens and global cognitive function in postmenopausal women: Women's health initiative memory study. *JAMA.*, 2004, 291, 2959-2968.

Gambrell, RD; Bagnell, CA; Greenblatt, RB. Role of oestrogens and progesterone in the etiology and prevention of endometrial cancer: a review. *Am J Obstet Gynecol*, 1983, 146, 696-707.

Garidou, L1; Laffont, S; Douin-Echinard, V; Coureau, C; Krust, A; Chambon, P; Guéry, JC. Estrogen receptor alpha signaling in inflammatory leukocytes is dispensable for 17beta-estradiol-mediated inhibition of experimental autoimmune encephalomyelitis. *J Immunol*, 2004, 173, 2435-2442.

Ghisletti, S; Meda, C; Maggi, A; Vegeto, E. 17beta-estradiol inhibits inflammatory gene expression by controlling NF-κB intracellular localization. *Mol Cell Biol*, 2005, 25, 2957-2968.

Guo, J; Krause, DN; Horne, J; Weiss, JH; Li, X; Duckles, SP. Oestrogen-receptor-mediated protection of cerebral endothelial cell viability and mitochondrial function after ischemic insult in vitro. *J Cereb Blood Flow Metab*, 2010, 3, 545-554.

Harris, HA; Albert, LM; Leathurby, Y; Malamas, MS; Mewshaw, RE; Miller, CP; Kharode, YP; Marzolf, J; Komm, BS; Winneker, RC; Frail, DE; Henderson, RA; Zhu, Y; Keith, JC. Evaluation of an estrogen receptor-beta agonist in animal models of human disease. *Endocrinology*, 2003, 144, 4241-4249.

Hickman, SE; Allison, EK; Khoury JE. Microglial dysfunction and defective beta-amyloid clearance pathways in aging Alzheimer's disease mice. *J Neurosci*, 2008, 8, 8354-8360.

Hilton, GD; Nunez, JL; Bambrick, L; Thompson, SM; McCarthy, MM. Glutamate-mediated excitotoxicity in neonatal hippocampal neurones is mediated by mGluR-induced release of Ca^{2+} from intracellular stores and is prevented by estradiol. *Eur J Neurosci*, 2006, 24, 3008-3016.

Hoffman, GE; Merchenthaler, I; Zup, SL. Neuroprotection by ovarian hormones in animal models of neurological disease. *Endocrine*, 2006, 29, 217-223.

Ibrahim, NK; Hortobagyi, GN. The evolving role of specific oestrogen receptor modulators (SERMs). *Surg Oncol*, 1999, 8, 103-123.

Ishihara, Y; Itoh, K; Ishida, A; Yamazaki, T. Selective estrogen-receptor modulators suppress microglial activation and neuronal cell death via an estrogen receptor-dependent pathway. *J Steroid Biochem Mol Biol*, 2015, 145, 85-93.

Jackson-Lewis, V; Przedborski, S. Protocol for the MPTP mouse model of Parkinson's disease. *Nat Protoc*, 2007, 2, 141-151.

Kim, HC; Bing, G; Kim, SJ; Jhoo, WK; Shin, EJ; Bok, Wie M; Ko, KH; Kim, WK; Flanders, KC; Choi, SG; Hong, JS. Kainate treatment alters TGF-β3 gene expression in the rat hippocampus. *Mol Brain Res*, 2002, 108, 60-70.

Kokiko, ON; Murashov, AK; Hoane, MR. Administration of raloxifene reduces sensorimotor and working memory deficits following traumatic brain injury. *Behav Brain Res*, 2006, 170, 233-240.

Kompoliti, K; Comella, CL; Jaglin, JA; Leurgans, S; Raman, R; Goetz, CG. Menstrual-related changes in motoric function in women with Parkinson's disease. *Neurology*, 2000, 55, 1572-1575.

Liu, B; Dluzen, DE. Oestrogen and nigrostriatal dopaminergic neurodegeneration: animal models and clinical reports of Parkinson's disease. *Clin Exp Pharmacol Physiol*, 2007, 34, 555-565.

Maggi, A; Ciana, P; Belcredito, S; Vegeto, E. Estrogens in the nervous system: mechanisms and non-reproductive functions. *Annu Rev Physiol*, 2004, 66, 291–313.

Maggi, A; Ciana, P; Belcredito, S; Vegeto, E. Estrogens in the nervous system: mechanisms and non-reproductive functions. *Annu Rev Physiol*, 2004, 66, 291-313.

Marinova-Mutafchieva, L; Sadeghian, M; Broom, L; Davis, JB; Medhurst, AD; Dexter, DT. Relationship between microglial activation and dopaminergic neuronal loss in the substantia nigra: a time course study in a 6-hydroxydopamine model of Parkinson's disease. *J Neurochem*, 2009, 110, 966-975.

Mayer, LP; Pearsall, NA; Christian, PJ; Devine, PJ; Payne, M; Mc-Cuskey, MK; Marion, SL; Sipes, IG; Hoyer, PB. Long-term effects of ovarian follicular depletion in rats by 4-vinylcyclohexene diepoxide. *Reprod Toxicol*, 2002, 16, 775–781.

McDermott, JL; Liu, B; Dluzen, DE. Sex differences and effects of estrogen on dopamine and DOPAC release from the striatum of male and female CD-1 mice. *Exp Neurol*, 1994, 125, 306-311.

Mitra, SW; Hoskin, E; Yudkovitz, J; Pear, L; Wilkinson, HA; Hayashi, S; Pfaff, DW; Ogawa, S; Rohrer, SP; Schaeffer, JM; McEwen, BS; Alves, SE. Immunolocalization of estrogen receptor β in the mouse brain: Comparison with estrogen receptor α. *Endocrinology*, 2003, 144, 2055-2067.

Morale, MC; Serra, PA; L'Episcopo, F; Tirolo, C; Caniglia, S; Testa, N; Gennuso, F; Giaquinta, G; Rocchitta, G; Desole, MS; Miele, E; Marchetti, B. Estrogen, neuroinflammation and neuroprotection in Parkinson's disease: glia dictates resistance versus vulnerability to neurodegeneration. *Neuroscience*, 2006, 138, 869-878.

Morales, LBJ; Loo, KK; Liu, HB; Peterson, C; Tiwari-Woodruff, S; Voskuhl, RR. Treatment with an estrogen receptor α ligand is neuroprotective in experimental autoimmune encephalomyelitis. *J Neurosci*, 2006, 26, 6823-6833.

Morissette, M; Di Paolo, T. Effect of chronic estradiol and progesterone treatments of ovariectomized rats on brain dopamine uptake sites. *J Neurochem*, 1993, 60, 1876-1883.

Najjar, S; Pearlman, DM; Alper, K; Najjar, A; Devinsky, O. Neuroinflammation and psychiatric illness. *J Neuroinflammation*, 2013, 10, 43.

Nilsson, S; Gustafsson, JA. Estrogen receptors: therapies targeted to receptor subtypes. *Clin Pharmacol Ther*, 2011, 89, 44-55.

Nilsson, S; Makela, S; Treuter, E; Tujague, M; Thomsen, J; Andersson, G; Enmark, E; Pettersson, K; Warner, M; Gustafsson, JA. Mechanisms of estrogen action. *Physiol Rev*, 2001, 81, 1535-1565.

Polanczyk, MJ; Hopke, C; Huan, J; Vandenbark, AA; Offner, H. Enhanced FoxP3 expression and Treg cell function in pregnant and estrogen-treated mice. *J Neuroimmunol*, 2005, 170, 85-92.

Pozzi, S; Benedusi, V; Maggi, A; Vegeto, E. Estrogen action in neuroprotection and brain inflammation. *Ann N Y Acad Sci*, 2006, 1089, 302-323.

Rapp, S; Espeland, M; Shumaker, S; Henderson, V; Brunner, R; Manson, J; Gass, M; Stefanick, M; Lane, D; Hays, J; Johnson, K; Coker, L; Dailey, M; Bowen, D. Effect of estrogen plus progestin on global cognitive function in postmenopausal women: The women's health initiative memory study: A randomized controlled trial. *JAMA*, 2003, 289, 2663-2672.

Reddy DS. The role of neurosteroids in the pathophysiology and treatment of catamenial epilepsy. *Epilepsy Res*, 2009, 85, 1-30.

Rocca, WA; Bower, JH; Maraganore, DM; Ahlskog, JE; Grossardt, BR; de Andrade, M; Melton, LJ. 3rd. Increased risk of cognitive impairment or dementia in women who underwent oophorectomy before menopause. *Neurology*, 2007, 69, 1074-1083.

Russo, J; Irma, H. The role of oestrogen in the initiation of breast cancer. *J Steroid Biochem Mol Biol*, 2006, 102, 89-96.

Saunders-Pullman, R; Gordon-Elliot, J; Parides, M; Fahn, S; Saunders, HR; Bressman, S. The effect of estrogen replacement on early replacement on early Parkinson's disease. *Neurology*, 1999, 52, 1417-1421.

Scharfman, HE; Malthankar-Phatak, GH; Friedman, D; Pearce, PP; McCloskey, DP; Harden, CL; Maclusky, NJ. A rat model of epilepsy in women: a tool to study physiological interactions between endocrine systems and seizures. *Endocrinology*, 2009, 150, 4437-4442.

Schauwecker, PE; Wood, RI; Lorenzana, A. Neuroprotection against excitotoxic brain injury in mice after ovarian steroid depletion. *Brain Res*, 2009, 1265, 37-46.

Subramanian, S; Matejuk, A; Zamora, A; Vandenbark, AA; Offner, H. Oral feeding with ethinyl estradiol suppresses and treats experimental autoimmune encephalomyelitis in SJL mice and inhibits the recruitment of inflammatory cells into the central nervous system. *J Immunol*, 2003, 170, 1548-1555.

Tolson, D; Fleming, V; Schartau E. Coping with menstruation: understanding the needs of women with Parkinson's disease. *J Adv Nurs*, 2002, 40, 513-521.

Tripanichkul, W; Sripanichkulchai, K; Finkelstein, S. Estrogen down-regulates glial activation in male mice following 1-methyl-4-phenyl-1,2,3,6-tetrahydropyridine intoxication. *Brain Res.*, 2006, 1084, 28-37.

Tsang, KL; Ho, SL; Lo, SK. Estrogen improves motor disability in parkinsonian postmenopausal women with motor fluctuations. *Neurology*, 2000, 54, 2292-2298.

Vegeto, E; Belcredito, S; Etteri, S; Ghisletti, S; Brusadelli, A; Meda, C; Krust, A; Dupont, S; Ciana, P; Chambon, P; Maggi, A. Estrogen receptor-alpha mediates the brain antiinflammatory activity of estradiol. *Proc Natl Acad Sci USA*, 2003, 100, 9614-9619.

Vegeto, E; Belcredito, S; Ghisletti, S; Meda, C; Etteri, S; Maggi, A. The endogenous estrogen status regulates microglia reactivity in animal models of neuroinflammation. *Endocrinol*, 2006, 147, 2263-2272.

Vegeto, E; Benedusi Maggi, A. Estrogen anti-inflammatory activity in brain: a therapeutic opportunity for menopause and neurodegenerative diseases. *Front Neuroendocrinol*, 2008, 29, 507-519.

Vegeto, E; Bonincontro, C; Pollio, G; Sala, A; Viappiani, S; Nardi, F; Brusadelli, A; Viviani, B; Ciana, P; Maggi, A. Estrogen prevents the lipopolysaccharide-induced inflammatory response in microglia. *J Neurosci*, 2001, 21, 1809-1818.

Vest, RS; Pike, CJ. Gender, sex steroid hormones, and Alzheimer's disease. *Horm Behav*, 2013, 63, 301-307.

Wang, YC; Lin, S; Yang, QW. Toll-like receptors in cerebral ischemic inflammatory injury. *J Neuroinflammation*, 2011, 8, 134.

Wynn, DR; Rodriguez, M; O'Fallon, WM; Kurland, LT. A reappraisal of the epidemiology of multiple sclerosis in Olmsted County, Minnesota. *Neurology*, 1990, 40, 780-786.

Xanthos, DN; Sandkuhler, J. Neurogenic neuroinflammation: inflammatory CNS reactions in response to neuronal activity, nature reviews. *Neuroscience*, 2014, 15, 43-53.

Xu, H; Gouras, GK; Greenfield, JP; Vincent, B; Naslund, J; Mazzarelli, L; Fried, G; Jovanovic, JN; Seeger, M; Relkin, NR; Liao, F; Checler, F; Buxbaum, JD; Chait, BT; Thinakaran, G; Sisodia, SS; Wang, R; Greengard, P; Gandy, S. Estrogen reduces neuronal generation of Alzheimer beta-amyloid peptides. *Nat Med*, 1998, 4, 447-451.

Yue, X; Lu, M; Lavcaster, T; Cao, P; Hnda, SI; Staufenbiel, M; Harada, N; Zhong, Z; Shen, Y; Li, R. Brain estrogen deficiency accelerates Abeta plaque formation in an Alzheimer's disease animal model. *Proc Natl Acad Sci USA*, 2005, 102, 19198-19203.

Xing, B; Xin, T; Hunter, RL; Bing, G. Pioglitazone inhibition of lipopolysaccharide-induced nitric oxide synthase is associated with altered activity of p38 MAP kinase and PI3K/Akt. *J Neuroinflammation*, 2008, 5, 4.

Zhao, L; O'Neill, K; Brinton, RD. Selective estrogen receptor modulators (SERMs) for the brain: current status and remaining challenges for developing NeuroSERMs. *Brain Res Rev*, 2005, 49, 472-493.

In: Neuroinflammation in Disease
Editor: Rebecca K. Dawson

ISBN: 978-1-63483-389-9
© 2015 Nova Science Publishers, Inc.

Chapter III

Dynamics of Establishment of Proinflammation As Signature Perivascular Injury in Multiple Sclerosis Neuroparenchyma

*Lawrence M. Agius**
Tal-Virtu, Rabat, Malta
Department of Pathology, Mater Dei Hospital,
University of Malta, Medical School, Msida, Malta

Abstract

Dynamics of progression in MS patients are indices of reference of an essential establishment of the disease process within contexts of proinflammatory reactivity and interactivity of an activated endothelial cell bed that perfuses the CNS parenchyma. The specific character of the activation of endothelial cells incorporates correlates of dynamic turnover and loss of myelin in plaques that persistently expand in a relapsing/ recurring manner. The inclusive phenomenon of endothelial cell response and injury calls, into operative distribution, lesions that comprise both

* Corresponding author: Telephone: (Home): 356-21451752, (Work): 356-2545-6444, Fax : 356-2545-6449, Email: lawrence.agius@um.edu.mt, lawrence.agius@gov.mt.

edema and ischemia within the individual MS plaque. It is such phenomenon of inclusive establishment of the initial microvascular injury that persists in terms of specific activation states of the endothelial cells lining post-capillary venules and capillaries of the cerebrovasculature.

Introduction

Cytokine and chemokine systems constitutively implicate targeted lymphocytes in many instances of neuroinflammation. As such, the evolutionary course of injury to neurons and brain parenchyma comprises a series of synergistically operative cascades that further involve targeting and agonist interactions. Matrix Metalloproteinases appear pathogenetically implicated in acute neuroinflammation [1]. The biology of neuroinflammatory processes is often in the form of exacerbations and remissions as noted clinically in many of the patients suffering from multiple sclerosis. There is further evidence to indicate the acute operative maintenance of an immuno-logic equilibrium particularly implicating both proinflammatory and also suppressive anti-inflammatory cytokines.

The significance of a reactive milieu for further promotion and exacerbation of neuroinflammation appears to concentrate or focus mainly within the perivascular regions of the neuro-environment. Posttranscriptional regulation of MMP2 and MMP9 expression specifies low gelatinase activity in the CNS and lymphocytes [2]. As such, the progression of spread of the proinflammatory agonists appears to evolve in terms of an essential imbalance between agonists such as tumor necrosis factor alpha and Interleukin I, on the one hand, and immunosuppressants such as transforming growth factor beta and Interleukins 4 and 10.

Proinflammation

The implications of an essential proinflammatory process appears to be suggestive of a self-established propensity for the institution of reactive phenomena within systems Lof plasticity and reactivity processes of the constitutive parametric evolution of agonist and parenchymal activity. Immune responses may be triggered by misfolded and aggregated proteins and cell specific stimuli [3].

Systems of establishment of multiple plaque formation arise inherently as processes of self-promoting inflammatory reactivity within the central nervous system.

It is significant to consider the disease course in these patients as a parameter of compounding influence within set patterns of action and reaction of cytokines and chemokines.

The perivascular inclusion of dynamic imbalance of promotional agonist action specifies, in turn, the incremental onset and further development of autoreactive T lymphocytes in the promoted cascades of pathway events. Multiple genetic risk loci have been identified in multiple sclerosis [4]

Targeting Events in MS

It would appear that the influences of targeting events are further amplified within the perivascular regions of the neuroparenchyma. In such manner, the true identifiable origins of neuro-reactive changes are originally developed around foci of increased permeability status of the blood-brain barrier. In such manner, constitutional facilitation of incremental and recurring proinflammatory processes are substantially self-promoting as evidenced by persistent susceptibility to future disease attacks in patients with multiple sclerosis. It is within such conceptual limits of confined perivascular spaces that the neuroinflammation further augments agonist-induced damage to myelin sheaths and neuronal loss in patients with established neuro-inflammation. The function of the blood-brain barrier is critical in this regard [5]. It is relative to such self-promoted facilitation and susceptibility to injury of the neuroparenchyma that the central role of perivascular activity identifies and ensures a persistence of proinflammatory activity of the disease process within the brain and spinal cord, in general terms, and particularly in patients suffering from multiple sclerosis. Systemic inflammation may often be implicated in the flaring up of symptoms in neurodegenerative disease [6]. It is in such terms that ischemia may prove a primary inducement for the proinflammatory agonists in patients that suffer from repeated episodes of demyelination in multiple sclerosis.

Dynamics of infiltrative components constitute both lymphocytes and macrophages in a manner that promotes microglial participation in subsequent reactivity.

It is in the real terms of such inflammatory plasticity that neuro-inflammation would implicate a valid contributory series of roles in both neuronal loss and active cellular degeneration. On the other hand, Natural killer cell subsets do not increase uniformly in all neuroinflammaory disorders [7], and may be involved in some cases in combating CNS immune activation.

Neuroparenchymal Dynamics

It would further appear that dynamic turnover specifies the true natural role of immune responses within the neuroparenchyma. Further to such establishment of the immune response there develops a system series of promotional progression that evolves as an essential component of the initial establishment of reactivity of the inflammation within the central nervous system. Precise identification of site and role of the pathogenetic factors is crucial [8].

Equilibrating dynamics of positively promoting and negatively suppressive dynamics would appear to underlie an essential susceptibility to injury within the inflammatory milieu of agonist action in particular. Tumor Necrosis Factor may help protect against neuroinflammation [9].

Indeed, dimensions of demyelinating foci would indeed progress as extensions both morphologically and dysfunctionally of the perivascular spaces of the brain and spinal cord . Restricted cell survival renewal and limited regenerativity ability render neural parenchyma expremely susceptible to injury by neuroinflammation [10]. The differential establishing dynamics of incremental activity influence the process of repeated susceptibility injury to such perivascular spaces in the central nervous system in multiple sclerosis patients. Further to such perivascular inflammatory reactivity a potentially identifiable profile of promotional susceptibility incorporates regions of the essential signature of disease pathogenesis in multiple sclerosis. Establishment of disease dynamics constitutes core processes of persistence and recurrence of demyelinating plaques in furthering the evolutionary character of the proinflammatory process. Semaphorin 7A and ala-Beta-his-dipeptidase may constitute CSF biomarkers in clinically definite MS conversion [11].

Neuroinflammation

In terms that operatively define neuroinflammation in patients with multiple sclerosis there evolves the establishment disease stage in further defining the nature of the multiple sclerosis pathogenic profile.

The disease process signature is the establishment of a proinflammatory susceptibility as confirmed and further propagated by the perivascular dynamics of interaction of agonists and inhibitors of the immune reactivity. Anti-inflammatory CD4(+) T cell subsets may delay the process of neurodegeneration [12].

The real formulation of multiple sclerosis involvement in a given patient is paramount dynamics of an injury constituted by the subsequent establishment of the immune response within the central nervous system.

Systems of promotion of venular and capillary permeability increases form a pathobiologic basis for the ingress of inflammatory cells and cytokine/chemokine molecules within the multiple sclerosis brain and spinal cord. J2 prostaglandins in particular are implicated in neuronal dysfunction induced by proinflammation [13]. Indeed, the molecular arrangements with positivity of these proinflammatory elements are characteristic of the demyelinating plaques in multiple sclerosis patients. The particular presence of tumor necrosis alpha and Interleukin I indicate also an inherent susceptibility for necrosis due to ischemia of the lesions. Such susceptibility may very well arise due to the progression of proinflammatory events affecting the microcirculation supplying the neuro-parenchyma. Additional susceptibility arises with the onset of progressive permeability of the cerebrovasculature leading to cerebral and spinal edema of the parenchyma [14].

Susceptibility Dynamics

Multiple sclerosis would appear to significantly implicate a series of compounding susceptibilities that arise within the context of an increased vascular permeability based on the opening of the junctional complexes. Such phenomenon includes a resulting lesion and activation of endothelial cells.

Brain miR-146a appears to inhibit NF-kB in the cerebral endothelial cells by inducing suppression of leukocyte adhesion during neuroinflammatory disorders [15].

The role of such cells implicates a loss of mitochondria and an increase in transcytotic transport with excess cytoplasmic vesicle formation within the endothelial cells.

In a significant manner, the essential state of activation of endothelial cells profoundly influences the course dynamics of the progressively persistent course of multiple sclerosis. Nonconventional MRI biomarkers are potentially especially useful for imaging the normal appearing brain parenchyma in multiple sclerosis [16].

Proliferation of astrocytes appears to constitute an essential correlate that results from dynamics of repetitive episodes of increased vascular permeability in the region of involvement of demyelination of the multiple sclerosis plaque.

This form of susceptibility itself subsequently precipitates further increases in microvascular permeability with the consequence of positive feedback events in the progression of plaque demyelination. STAT 5 is required for regulatory T helper-cell generation and immune suppression [17].

In a real sense, the dynamics of plaque demyelination appear to constitute relative consequences of the endothelial cell activation cycles within the CNS microvasculature, in a specific manner, that correlates increased permeability of the venular/capillary wall with essential ischemia and edema of the inflammatory demyelination substrate of the individual plaques. MMP2 and MMP9 cleave blood brain barrier beta-dystrophin to thus break down the parenchymal basement membrane [18].

Demyelination

Within the complex interactivities of progressive demyelination in multiple sclerosis there would evolve an established series of sequential events in the form of involvement of endothelial cells. Such pathogenetic activation of the microvasculature determines the persistent establishment of the proinflammatory activity and response of the dynamic demyelination and of subsequent attempts at remyelination of the plaque lesions.

Developmental endothelial locus-1 acts homeostatically to limit neuroinflammation [19].

Lesioned increments of parametric influence in blood-brain barrier permeability come to actively constitute the biologic stratum for a progressive disease course dominated by initial establishment of proinflammation within the endothelial cells lining the CNS microvasculature. Some hedgehog released by astrocytes helps maintain blood-brain barrier integrity [20].

As a consequence, a multitude of pathologic events contribute to signature promotion that earmarks the progression of plaque demyelination as cyclical predominance and as involvement of hypertrophic astrogliosis within the regions of individual plaques. Multiple substrates for transglutaminases implicate catalysis of protein crosslinking in neuroinflammation [21].

Positive feed- back pathways are essential targeting events that transform the dynamics of endothelial cell activation systems. Indeed, the proinflammatory molecular events within the MS microvasculature are themselves mechanisms of targeting of the individual endothelial cells themselves.

Plaque demyelination arises as expression of aberrant profiles of activation of the individual endothelial cells that control/decontrol systems of susceptibility within the CNS microvasculature. However, Epstein-Barr virus-specific intrathecal synthesis of oligoclonal IGG may only be a nonspecific component of humoral polyreactivity in chronic neuroinflammatory states [22].

Plaque Ischemia and Edema

Turn-over events of targeting endothelial cells characterize specific attributes of the activation of the lining vascular wall in the profile accommodation of system establishment that marks proinflammation and blood flow defects of the microcirculation. Indeed, ischemia of progressively demyelinating plaques includes the correlating astrogliosis and a system susceptibility of complement and coagulation cascades within regions of activated micro-vasculature.

Immunologic responses appear to induce disease progression in neurodegeneration in general [23].

An essential profile understanding of disease dynamics as progressive plaque demyelination includes essential interactivities with involvement of increased microvascular permeability within specific dynamics of the activation of lining endothelial cells of the post-capillary venules in particular. Capillaries participate essentially as promotional profile susceptibility that specifies the signature lesion within activated endothelial cells constituting the CNS microvasculature. In such manner, derivative events result in demyelination of plaques that actively constitutes foci of ischemia and edema of the myelin sheath of axons traversing such MS plaques.

Conclusion

The distributional susceptibilities to a signature lesion within individually activated endothelial cells of the MS microvasculature correlate with essential promotion of cytokine/chemokine interactivities of the specific pathogenetic pathways of transcytotic and of junctional complex permeability and pore formation of such vascular components. Increments for the initial establishment of the primary lesion in MS patients actively promote the decisive proinflammatory events that specify dynamics of the activated status of the endothelial cells.

Within the substantial promotion of incremental lesion creation there are the specific profile dynamics of inclusive phenomena of vascular hyper-permeability and edema formation within the MS plaques.

Derivative promotion of such events of susceptibility comes to specify the further increments in progression of demyelination. Such demyelination includes the persistence of performance of MS plaques within contexts of further progressive myelin loss.

References

[1] Ljukisavljevic, C; Stojanovic, I; Basic, J; Vojinovic, S; Stojanov, C; Djordjevic, G; et al. "The role of matrix metalloproteinase 3 and 9 in the pathogenesis of Acute Neuroinflammation. Implications for disease modifying therapy." *J. Mol. Neurosci*, 2015 Feb 22.

[2] Petkovic, F; Zivanovic, J; Blazevski, J; Timolijevic, G; Momcilovic, M; Stanojevic, Z; et al. "Activity; but not mRNA expression of gelatinases correlates with susceptibility to experimental autoimmune encephalomyelitis" *Neuroscience*, 2015 Feb 18, 292C, 1-13.

[3] Anderson, KM; Olson, KE; Estes, KA; Flanagan, K; Gendelman, HE; Mosley, RL. "Dual destructive and protective roles of adaptive immunity in neurodegenerative disorders" *Transl Neurodegener*, 2014 Nov 13, 3(1), 25.

[4]   Hoppmann, N; Graetz, C; Paterka, M; Poisa-Beiro, L; Larochelle, C; Hasan, M; et al. "New candidates of CD4 T cell pathogenecity in experimental neuroinflammation and multiple sclerosis" *Brain*, 2015 Feb 9.

[5]   Gauberti, M; Montagne, A; Quenault A; Vivien, D. "Molecular magnetic resonance imaging of brain-immunointeractions" *Front Cell Neurosci*, 2014 Nov 27, 8, 389.

[6]   Murta, V; Farias, MI; Pitossi, FJ; Ferrari, CC. "Chronic systemic IL-1Beta exacerbates central neuroinflammation independently of the blood-brain barrier integrity" *J Neuroimmunol*, 2015 Jan 15, 278, 30-43.

[7]   Rodriquez-Martin, E; Picon, C; Costa-Frossard, L; Alenda, R; Sainz de la Maza, S; Roldan E; et al. "Natural killer cell subsets in cerebrospinal fluid of patients with multiple sclerosis" *Clin Exp Immuol*, 2015 Jan 7.

[8]   Ljubisavljevic, S. "Oxidative stress and neurobiology of demyelination" *Mol Neurobiol*, 2014 Dec 11.

[9]   Blazevski, J; Pelkovic, F; Momcilovic, M; Jeutic, B; Stojkovic, MM; Miljkovic, D. "Tumor necrosis factor stimulates expression of CXCL12 in astrocytes" *Immunobiology*, 2015 Jan 22.

[10]   Srinivasau, M; Lahiri, DK. "Significance of NF-kB as a pivotal therapeutic target in the neurodegenerative pathologies of Alzheimer's disease and multiple sclerosis" *Expert Opin Ther Targets*, 2015 Feb 4, 1-17.

[11]   Canto, E; Tintore, M; Villar, LM; Borras, E; Alvarez-Cermeno, JC; Chiva, C; et al. "Validation of semaphoring 1A and ala-Beta-his-dipeptidase as biomarkers associated with the conversion from clinically isolated syndrome to multiple sclerosis" *J Neuroinflammation*, 2014 Nov 13, 11, 181.

[12]   Gonzalez, H; Pacheco, R. "T-cell-mediated regulation of neuroinflammation involved in neurodegenerative disease" *J Neuroinflammation*, 2014 Dec 21 11L201.

[13]   Fiquelredo-Pereira, ME; Rockwell, P; Schmidt-Glenewinkel, T; Serrano, P. "Neuroinflammation and J2 prostglandins: linking impairment of the ubiquitin-proteasome pathway and mitochondria to neurodegeneration" *Front Mol Neurosci*, 2015 Jan 13, 7, 104.

[14]   Jonas, A; Thiem, S; Kuhlmann, T; Waginer, R; Aszodi, A; Novell, C; et al. "Axonally derived matrilin-2 induces proinflammatory responses that exacerbate autoimmune neuroinflammation" *J Clin Invest*, 2014 Nov, 124(11), 5042-56

[15] Wu, D; Cerutti, C; Lopez-Ramirez, MA; Pryce, G; King-Robson, J; Simpson, JE; et al. "Brain endothelial miR-146a negatively modulates T-cell adhesion through repressing multiple targets to inhibit NF-kB activation" *J Cereb Blood Flow Metab*, 2015 Mar, 35(3), 412-23.

[16] Londono, AC; Mora, CA. "Nonconventional MRI biomarkers for in vivo monitoring of pathogenesis in multiple sclerosis" *Neurol Neuroimmunol Neuroinflamm*, 2014 Nov 20, 1(4), e45

[17] Sheng, W; Yang, F; Zhu, Y; Yang, H; Low, PY; Kemeny, DM; et al. "Stat-5 programs a distinct subset of GM-CSF-producing T helper cells that is essential for autoimmune neuroinflammation" *Cell Res*, 2014 Dec, 24(12), 1387-402.

[18] Vandooren, J; Van Damme, J; Opdenakker, G. "On the structure and functions of gelatinase B/matrix Metalloproteinase-9 in neuroinflammation" *Prog Brain Res*, 2014, 193-206.

[19] Choi, EY; Lim, JH; Neuwirth, A; Economopoulou, M; Chatzigeorgiou, A; Chung, K; et al. "Developmental endothelial locus-1 is a homeostatic factor in the central nervous system limiting neuroinflammation and demyelination" *Mol Psychiatry*, 2014 Nov 11

[20] Wang, Y; Jin, S; Sonobe, Y; Cheng, Y; Horinchi, H; parajuli, B; et al. "Interleukin-1B induces blood brain barrier disruption by downregulating Soni Hedgehog in astrocytes' *PLos One*, 2014 Oct 14, 9(10)

[21] Ientile, R; Curro, M; Caccamo, D. "Transglutaminase 2 and neuroinflammation" *Amino Acids*, 2015 Jan, 47(1), 19-26.

[22] Castellazzi, M; Contini, C; Tamborino, C; Fasolo, F; Roversi, G; Seraceni, S; et al. "Epstein-Barr virus-specific intrathecal oligoclonal IgG production in relapsing-remitting multiple sclerosis is limited to a subset of patients and is composed of low-affinity antibodies" *J Neuroinflammation*, 2014 Nov 13, 11(1), 188.

[23] Sloeck, K; Schmitz, M; Ebert, E; Schmidt, C; Zerr, I. "Immune responses in rapidly progressive dementia: a comparative study of neuroinflammatory markers in Creutzfeldt-Jakob disease Alzheimer's disease and multiple sclerosis" *J Neuroinflammation*, 2014 Oct 15, 11(1), 170

Index

F

G

H

I

N

O